Essential Cardiac Catheterization

Essential Cardiac Catheterization

Supported by an educational grant
from **Medtronic**

Rob Butler
Consultant Cardiologist, Department of Cardiology,
City General Hospital, University Hospital of North
Staffordshire, Stoke on Trent, UK

Mark Gunning
Consultant Cardiologist, Department of Cardiology,
City General Hospital, University Hospital of North
Staffordshire, Stoke on Trent, UK

James Nolan
Consultant Cardiologist, Department of Cardiology,
City General Hospital, University Hospital of North
Staffordshire, Stoke on Trent, UK

Hodder Arnold

A MEMBER OF THE HODDER HEADLINE GROUP

First published in Great Britain in 2007 by
Hodder Arnold, an imprint of Hodder Education and a member of the
Hodder Headline Group,
338 Euston Road, London NW1 3BH

http://www.hoddereducation.com

198 Madison Avenue, New York, NY10016
Oxford is a registered trademark of Oxford University Press

Whilst the advice and information in this book are believed to be true and accurate at the date
of going to press, neither the author[s] nor the publisher can accept any legal responsibility or
liability for any errors or omissions that may be made. In particular, (but without limiting the
generality of the preceding disclaimer) every effort has been made to check drug dosages;
however it is still possible that errors have been missed. Furthermore, dosage schedules are
constantly being revised and new side-effects recognized. For these reasons the reader is
strongly urged to consult the drug companies' printed instructions before administering any of
the drugs recommended in this book.

British Library Cataloguing in Publication Data
A catalogue record for this book is available from the British Library

Library of Congress Cataloging-in-Publication Data
A catalog record for this book is available from the Library of Congress

ISBN   978-0-340-88735-6

1 2 3 4 5 6 7 8 9 10

Commissioning Editor:	Philip Shaw
Project Editor:	Heather Fyfe
Production Controller:	Karen Tate
Cover Design:	Sarah Rees

Typeset in [10/12 Minion] by Charon Tec Ltd (A Macmillan Company), Chennai, India
www.charontec.com
Printed and bound in Italy

What do you think about this book? Or any other Hodder Arnold title?
Please visit our website www.hoddereducation.com

Contents

Preface

Catheter laboratory training as a junior cardiologist is an exciting time, accompanied by a feeling of finally undertaking something exclusive to cardiologists. Consequently, it is highly valued amongst trainees, particularly early on. In this climate of increased accountability and vigilance, the times of being left to learn by osmosis, supervised essentially by your peers have gone. However the learning process is experience based; you learn on the cases that are available to you with guidance from more senior trainees and teaching by cardiologists. Structured programmes for catheter lab training are not fully developed in the UK.

The basic facts needed by a trainee are often not formally set out, and the rapidly evolving and very useful change in access route from brachial or femoral to radial artery is not covered in many centres. A compact text would be useful for core information and for reference in more esoteric investigations during training.

Between us we hope to have created a useful resource for the catheter lab trainee, whatever their subspecialty interest in cardiology eventually proves to be.

Rob Butler
Mark Gunning
Jim Nolan

Acknowledgements

We are grateful to our wives and partners for the support given during the preparation of this text.

The assistance of many colleagues, consultant and technical, has also been invaluable, providing DICOM images and allowing pictures to be taken in the cath lab to illustrate the text.

An introduction to the catheter laboratory: key responsibilities and patient preparation

1

Introduction

Coronary angiography began over 150 years ago, in 1844, when Claude Bernard catheterized a horse. Then in the 1920s, Werner Forssmann, a trainee surgeon in Germany, became the first human subject when he catheterized himself, documenting correct catheter placement by walking to the radiology department for a confirmatory plain film. Forssmann went on to share the Nobel Prize for Medicine in 1956 with Andre Cournand and Dickinson Richards for their contributions to the development of cardiac catheterization.

In 1930 O. Klein reported a series of right heart studies to measure cardiac output by the Fick principle. Cournand and Richards further developed the technique in the 1940s. From this time advances were made quickly, and the technique of cardiac catheterization became widely available worldwide (Table 1.1).

Since these early days the diagnostic angiographic equipment we use today has evolved more gradually. Major technological advances have come mainly from advances in material sciences. Better vascular access site technology, better tolerated contrast agents, more flexible and softer tipped catheters with larger lumens but smaller external calibre make the diagnostic angiogram of the twenty-first century a completely different clinical experience for the doctor and patient compared with earlier experience. Perhaps the biggest change over the last 10 years has been the move from cine film-based archiving systems to digital storage media and the gradual transition back to using upper limb access sites for cardiac catheterization.

The clinical need for cardiac catheterization has also grown dramatically, driven in part by the ease, reliability and relatively low risk of the procedure, but also by the enormous medical and financial burden of coronary artery disease. Twenty or thirty years ago, although the

Table 1.1 Technical advances in cardiac catheterization

Date	Technical advance
1950	Retrograde left heart catheter
1953	Seldinger technique
1959	Trans-septal puncture and selective coronary angiography
1967	Percutaneous selective angiography
1970s	Brachial route pioneered – Mason Sones
1970s	Preformed femoral catheters – Drs Judkins and Amplatz

angiographic information was available, therapeutic options were relatively restricted. However, with advances in cardiac surgical techniques, surgically based revascularization strategies have become available, and cardiology and cardiac surgery have began to flourish. Until recently, although cardiologists were in a key position to provide surgeons with cases, they had no techniques available to treat coronary disease themselves other than by drug therapy. The cardiac surgeon was king. Now, the rapid evolution of catheter-based therapies for coronary intervention and electrophysiology has provided a huge impetus for the use of cardiac catheterization as the 'gold standard' imaging technique for coronary arteries and has shifted the balance of power back towards cardiology. So much so that in the UK, for example, cardiac surgery is in decline.

The future of the catheter lab-based cardiologist is perhaps more uncertain, and the developing role of cardiac magnetic resonance (CMR) or computerized tomography (CT)-based diagnostic cardiology remains an exciting unknown. However, for the foreseeable future, the catheter lab skills for angiography will be the basis for diagnosis and also for those skills required for more definitive therapies such as percutaneous intervention and electrophysiology (Figure 1.1).

The role of cardiac catheterization and coronary angiography

Correct terminology is important to avoid confusion. Two terms, cardiac catheterization and coronary angiography, are often used interchangeably, but in fact they are subtly different. Within this text we make the following distinctions:

- *Cardiac catheterization*: This is an umbrella term for all aspects of right and left heart catheterization from any percutaneous route.
- *Coronary angiography*: This term is used only to indicate selective intubation and visualization of a coronary artery.
- *Non-coronary angiography*: In this book the only non-coronary angiography will be aortography, pulmonary and renal angiography.

Right heart studies are performed as isolated studies in less than 1 per cent of catheter lab cases in our unit. Combined right and left heart studies take up about 7 per cent of studies. The remainder are left heart catheterization procedures – usually a combination of coronary angiography and left ventriculography.

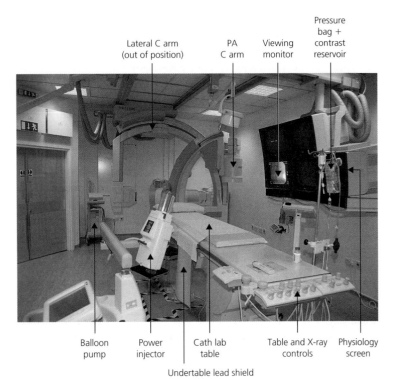

Lateral C arm (out of position) — PA C arm — Viewing monitor — Pressure bag + contrast reservoir

Balloon pump — Power injector — Cath lab table — Table and X-ray controls — Physiology screen

Undertable lead shield

Figure 1.1   Biplane catheter laboratory.

The role of right heart studies is discussed more fully in Chapter 6, but in essence this procedure gives information regarding intracardiac pressures, cardiac output, systemic vascular resistance and facilitates the assessment of intracardiac shunts.

Left heart studies provide information regarding left ventricular function, aortic dimension, aortic valve and left ventricular outflow tract gradients and the severity of aortic and mitral regurgitation. Left heart studies usually also provide images of the coronary arteries and all of their attendant diseases.

Coronary atheroma generates the bulk of the work of worldwide catheter labs and coronary angiography is ideally placed to accurately identify obstructive atheromatous plaque disease, coronary dissection, thrombus, spasm, myocardial bridging, calcification and aneurysms. The growing availability of the technique means that it is ideally placed to assess coronary disease in a variety of clinical scenarios: stable angina, unstable angina and acute myocardial infarction.

Cardiac catheterization provides critical information in a timely and essentially safe manner. It remains a fresh and exciting technique, which continues on occasion to tax even the most experienced cardiologist.

Key catheter laboratory information

Personal and institutional skill levels

There are a number of issues regarding angiographic training and maintaining competency once trained. The cardiac catheterization laboratory has a role as an institution in maintaining quality control of equipment, training and supervision. This function is often overlooked by the trainee as being largely irrelevant to their own day-to-day practice, but is critical in managing the safe investigation of heart disease.

The institution that undertakes angiography should have rapid access to a number of key supporting clinical services (Table 1.2). Although angiography is now a relatively low risk procedure, cases still develop complications, some of which need rapid diagnosis and urgent treatment. There is a move worldwide towards catheter labs being located in district/non-tertiary hospitals. This in itself is not an issue, as long as workable plans are made to manage these complications, some of which can be rapid in onset and of deadly consequence.

What logically follows on from this is the appropriate case selection in the various types of catheter lab: full tertiary centre, district hospital and mobile/free standing units which visit some hospitals. Consensus would

Table 1.2   Ideal speciality support for the cardiac catheterization lab

Additional speciality support
Cardiac surgery
Coronary and intensive care units
Vascular surgery
Nephrology
Neurology
Haematology/blood bank services
Imaging services (CT, MRI and ultrasound)
Adapted from ACC/SCA&I Expert Consensus Document on Cath Lab Standards [1].

Table 1.3 Appropriate case mix in catheterization labs

	Contraindications
Non-tertiary centre	Age >75 years
	NYHA Class III or IV heart failure
	Acute, intermediate or high-risk ischaemic syndromes
	Recent myocardial infarction with postinfarction ischaemia
	Pulmonary oedema thought to be caused by ischaemia
	High likelihood of or known left main stem or severe multivessel coronary disease
	Severe valvular dysfunction, especially in the setting of depressed left ventricular performance
	Patients at increased risk for vascular complications
	Complex adult congenital heart disease
Freestanding laboratory	All of the above plus:
	No therapeutic procedures
	Patients at high risk due to the presence of comorbid conditions, including the need for anticoagulation therapy, poorly controlled hypertension or diabetes, contrast allergy or renal failure

Adapted from ACC/SCA&I Expert Consensus Document on Cath Lab Standards [1].

suggest that acute coronary syndromes, severe decompensated heart failure and other high-risk conditions should only be safely studied in a tertiary equivalent unit. The American College of Cardiology/Society for Cardiac Angiography and Interventions (ACC/SCA&I) goes further and suggests the restrictions listed in Table 1.3 on case mix in non-tertiary and mobile labs.

Personal competency

The current British guidelines for training in diagnostic angiography are set by the British Cardiac Society and the Specialty Advisory Committee in Cardiovascular Medicine of the Royal College of Physicians [2] (Box 1.1).

Although 250 cardiac catheterizations is a modest number, it is in keeping with the minimum required in the USA, where current basic training requires four months and 100 diagnostic catheters. Advanced catheter lab training requires 300 cases, with 200 as the primary operator. This equates to 400 cases with 200 as primary operator.

The difficulty is that this represents the minimum, and by no means necessarily equates with satisfactory technical competence. The relatively

> **Box 1.1** BCS/RCP diagnostic cardiology guidelines. Invasive and interventional cardiology: basic training [2]
>
> Proficiency is required in coronary arteriography and left and right heart catheterization. The speed with which people learn practical procedures varies considerably. The trainees will be regarded as proficient once the trainer considers that they can be left alone to perform routine cases quite safely and they have carried out the required number of investigations (200 coronary angiograms and 50 left and right heart catheterizations as the first or only operator). Furthermore the trainer must be satisfied that the trainee can interpret the results of such investigations accurately and reliably. The results should be analysed and the angiograms viewed with a senior colleague in a formal reporting session: this should involve discussion with cardiac surgeons as appropriate.

short training period may not be sufficient to see major anatomical variations, difficult cases and adequate exposure to infrequent but major complications, as well as the difficult-to-acquire skill of interpretation. Often it is the doctor whose aspiration is not to be based in the catheter lab the majority of time who manages to accrue the necessary 250 cases, but may then practice in the most exposed locations in district hospitals, with significantly less peer support.

It is important to gain as much experience as possible. Unbiased assessment of hand skills is necessary by experienced trainers to ensure that a trainee who lacks the degree of co-ordination necessary for cardiac catheterization is directed to an alternative subspecialization.

Indications for cardiac catheterization and coronary angiography

The indications for invasive investigation of the heart are many, and the list changes as new techniques arrive with a fanfare and retreat to find a smaller more sustainable niche (Table 1.4). Broadly, the role of right heart catheterization is diminishing, as echocardiography, CMR imaging and multislice CT develop. These techniques provide much better anatomical definition of the heart and great vessels.

The evolution of CMR with respect to right heart pathology is particularly interesting. Cardiac catheterization is excellent for pressure measurement and recording, as well as establishing cardiac output, and providing shunt information. On the other hand it is very poor at assessing right heart function because 2D projection hides so much of the useful information, given the right heart's awkward shape. CMR gives excellent anatomical detail and information regarding function. In addition it can also give an assessment of pressure gradients across valves, analogous to echocardiographic-derived Doppler velocity signals.

The bulk of the indications for invasive investigation of the heart are to diagnose and quantify the extent of occlusive coronary artery disease. This is essentially left heart catheterization – coronary and left ventricular angiography (Table 1.5).

Table 1.4   Broad indications for right heart assessment

Condition	Examples	
Valve disease	Mitral valve disease	Pulmonary hypertension on echo or poor pulmonary window on echocardiography
Congenital heart disease	Atrial septal defect, ventricular septal defect, etc.	Assessment of chamber size and shunt size
Ischaemic heart disease	Cardiogenic shock Right heart failure	
Hypotension	Septic shock	Assessment of systemic vascular resistance

Table 1.5   Indications for left heart catheterization

Condition	Examples	Highlighted at-risk groups
Ischaemic heart disease	Chest pain ?cause	Suspicious findings on non-invasive investigations such as exercise testing or radionucleotide imaging. Also to confirm the absence of coronary artery disease in the nuisance patient
	Stable angina	Severe or progressive symptoms of angina Positive non-invasive testing
	Acute coronary syndromes	Unstable or dynamic ECG changes Identifying appropriate patients for percutaneous or early surgical revascularization in non-ST elevation myocardial infarction
		Primary and rescue percutaneous intervention

(Continued)

Table 1.5 (*Continued*)

Condition	Examples	Highlighted at-risk groups
	Post revascularization chest pain	Recent percutaneous coronary intervention because of subacute thrombosis or abrupt vessel closure
		In stent restenosis with recurrence of chest pain
		Post coronary artery bypass grafting with high risk findings on non-invasive imaging
Valvular heart disease		Before valve surgery to assess need for surgical revascularization
Heart failure		Heart failure with angina Pre cardiac transplantation Heart failure post myocardial infarction

Contraindications to cardiac catheterization

The advisability of any test is dependent on weighing the risk and the benefit for each and every patient (Table 1.6). Each patient's current situation and pre-existing state of health varies so much that it is impossible to give hard and fast rules. However, there are a number of situations where the degree of arm twisting needed to force cardiac catheterization in a non-life threatening situation varies to a greater or lesser extent. Some of these will be addressed in this chapter as part of the strategy for minimizing the potential hazard of an angiographic procedure in at-risk/high-risk patients.

Selecting the patient for catheter lab investigation

Ischaemic heart disease

There are an increasing number of clinical scenarios when diagnostic angiography is required as part of the assessment of coronary artery disease (CAD), as the culture of cardiology and accessibility of catheter labs changes and improves. The previously used and often quite inflexible benchmarks, such as using the achievement of 6 min exercise on a standard Bruce protocol exercise tolerance test as a cut-off for the need for angiography, can be unhelpful. This strategy developed as much to

Table 1.6   Relative contraindications to cardiac catheterization

Increased bleeding diathesis
  Haemophilia
  Heparin
  Bivalirudin
  Warfarin
  Glycoprotein IIb–IIIa inhibitors
Severe heart failure
Renal failure
Previous contrast reaction
Agitated patient
Uncontrolled hypertension
Febrile illness
Drug toxicity
Stroke
Hypokalaemia

gatekeep access to angiography when it was a severely limited resource as to encourage it.

Indeed, we feel that angiography has a valuable role in excluding the presence of occlusive flow-limiting disease in some patient groups, even with a low pretest probability of having CAD. Being able to reassure the patient that the coronary arteries are angiographically normal can be very helpful in their management, reducing unnecessary admissions to hospital and patient anxiety.

A common concern is the cardiac catheterization list that seems to have a disproportionate number of normal patients, provoking the thought that you may be overinvestigating your patients. In a risk-free procedure this would not matter. However, every catheterization procedure increases the risk of a major adverse clinical event (i.e. death, stroke or myocardial infarction).

A number of historical sources place the expected number of normal procedures between 20 per cent and 27 per cent [3,4]. This suggests that between a fifth and a quarter of all cases should be normal, based on the pretest probability of disease and clinical acumen.

The selection of patients can be difficult, and it is almost impossible to write clear guidelines to cover all eventualities. However, some understanding of the non-invasive tests available and the impact that the pretest probability of disease has on the likelihood of ultimately having coronary disease is important to help select appropriate patients for angiography.

The aim of non-invasive testing is to substratify those deemed at intermediate risk, where low risk is <1 per cent risk of death, medium risk is 1–3 per cent risk of death and high risk is >3 per cent risk of death. Those with low risk probably do not warrant any investigation and those at high risk should proceed directly to invasive investigation (i.e. cardiac catheterization). Those who are at high risk, with an annual risk of death of >3 per cent, potentially gain substantial benefit from any resulting revascularization.

In the UK, there are three main tests currently available that allow non-invasive testing for CAD. These are:

- Exercise tolerance test
- Stress echocardiography
- Myocardial perfusion imaging.

Other tests, such as CMR imaging and positron emission tomography (PET) are not yet widely available.

EXERCISE TOLERANCE TESTING

The majority of exercise tolerance tests (ETTs) in the UK are performed using treadmills with online ECG analysis, following standard exercise protocols with a graded increase in workload (i.e. Bruce and modified Bruce). Previously, the cut-off for warranting invasive chest investigation with angiography was being able to perform <6 min of a Bruce protocol test (<12 min of modified Bruce) with chest pain or ECG changes >1 mm in two or more leads. The pretest probability markedly affects the outcome of the test (Table 1.7).

Patients with a low pretest probability are much more likely to have a false-positive exercise test, and therefore a positive test is unlikely to be helpful. Often you are then obliged to undertake a further confirmatory test, with additional risk to the patient and a low associated diagnostic yield. Similarly patients with a high pretest probability are likely to have CAD at angiography anyway, and the ETT has little additional diagnostic utility. These patients should probably proceed directly to angiography.

The role of ETT is in the discrimination of those subjects with an intermediate pretest probability. The presence of more than 1 mm of planar ST depression in two or more leads with chest pain and ECG changes is likely to predict the presence of CAD. If the baseline ECG is normal, then these changes are even more likely to represent true positives.

Table 1.7   Pretest probability and likelihood of coronary disease

		Typical angina	Effort-related pain	Atypical pain	Asymptomatic
30–39	Male	Intermediate	Intermediate	Low	Low
	Female	Intermediate	Low	Low	Low
40–49	Male	High	Intermediate	Intermediate	Low
	Female	Intermediate	Low	Low	Low
50–59	Male	High	Intermediate	Intermediate	Low
	Female	Intermediate	Intermediate	Low	Low
60–69	Male	High	Intermediate	Intermediate	Low
	Female	High	Intermediate	Intermediate	Low

Modified from ACC/AHA 2002 Guideline Update for Exercise Testing [5].
Prevalence of coronary artery disease: low <10%; intermediate 10–90%;
high >90%.

Lower specificity is seen in patients in whom false-positive results are more likely, such as those with valvular heart disease, left ventricular hypertrophy, resting ST depression, and patients taking digoxin. Similarly, accessory pathways such as in the Wolff–Parkinson–White syndrome and paced rhythms are more difficult to interpret.

Overall, ETT in patients without valvular heart disease, left ventricular hypertrophy, resting ST depression and digoxin effect had a sensitivity of 68 per cent, specificity of 77 per cent and a predictive accuracy of 73 per cent in a meta-analysis of 24 000 patients [6].

The role of beta-blockers in exercise testing has stimulated considerable debate. It is not necessary to routinely stop beta-blockers during an exercise test, as the diagnostic yield does not drop, although this remains standard practice in many cardiac units. Obviously the patient is unlikely to reach the same heart rate rise with beta-blockers on board, and this needs to be taken account of. It would be prudent to be aware of local practice to prevent conflict with colleagues.

ST elevation is very significant during an ETT, but is uncommon. However, if Q waves are present in the leads that demonstrate the ST–T elevation, then their significance is reduced. Some patients are unable to exercise and the yield of positive exercise tests with those patients is also high.

STRESS ECHOCARDIOGRAPHY

This procedure is increasingly available in the UK. The essence of the test is to compare areas of the heart before and after stress, and look for regional wall motion abnormalities, which suggest the presence of ischaemia. In patients with an intermediate/high pretest probability of CAD, exercise stress echocardiography has a sensitivity of 86 per cent, a specificity of 81 per cent, and an overall diagnostic accuracy of 85 per cent. The sensitivity and specificity in the presence of pharmacological stress is very similar. Stress is induced either by adrenergic stimulation, with agents such as dobutamine or arbutamine, or vasodilatation with agents such as dipyridamole or adenosine. Stress echocardiography is not recommended in patients with a low pretest probability of having CAD.

Stress echocardiography has a number of advantages over exercise testing by treadmill and realtime ECG monitoring. It may be better at picking up multivessel disease and left main stem disease and is significantly better at localizing ischaemia than standard treadmill testing. It has a role in patients in whom standard exercise testing is difficult to achieve or interpret, such as those with:

- valvular heart disease
- left ventricular hypertrophy
- resting ST depression
- taking digoxin
- Wolff–Parkinson–White syndrome
- paced rhythms.

However it is more time consuming than other techniques, and most echocardiography departments are severely under pressure with the demands for standard transthoracic echocardiography.

MYOCARDIAL PERFUSION IMAGING

This test has also been hampered by poor availability in the UK, but this situation is rapidly improving. Myocardial perfusion imaging with tracers such as thallium (Tl-201), technetium (Tc-99m-sestamibi and Tc-99m-tetrofosmin) all yield similar percentage sensitivities in the high 80s and specificities in the mid 70s.

The essence of the test is to stress the patient, either by treadmill testing or by pharmacological challenge, and to inject a gamma-emitting tracer, such as thallium or technetium. This will be taken up by areas of the heart that are perfused and gaps will appear in the resulting picture of myocardial perfusion indicating reduced flow, or scar and potential ischaemia. The heart is then allowed to rest and (in the case of technetium tracers) a second injection is administered. Infarcted areas will have a reduced/absent tracer uptake on both the stress and rest images, whereas ischaemic areas will demonstrate some recovery of tracer uptake on the rest images when compared with the stress images. Obviously normal perfusion will not demonstrate reduced tracer uptake on either rest or stress images.

Myocardial perfusion imaging has a number of advantages over treadmill testing insofar as it can identify the extent of previously infarcted myocardium, the amount of myocardium at risk and also the severity of perfusion impairment. It can also be used in patients with a contraindication to ETT and patients with ventricular pre-excitation left ventricular hypertrophy, who are taking digoxin therapy or have more than 1 mm ST depression.

It is less useful in certain other circumstances. Left bundle branch block and paced rhythms reduce the usefulness of the test and pharmacological stress needs to be performed with vasodilators rather than adrenergic agonists. Similarly, large breasts in women or severe obesity can cause artefacts which may be mistaken for ischaemia in the anterior wall. It is also more difficult to assess left main stem disease in a left dominant system. This is because myocardial perfusion imaging relies on differential tracer uptake. If the heart has a left dominant system, and hence all major territories are dependent on the left coronary artery, then left main stem disease can cause a global reduction in tracer uptake and be missed. Consequently, subjects who have symptoms consistent with left main stem disease probably should proceed directly to angiography.

One particularly useful strength of myocardial perfusion imaging is the ability to assess myocardial viability, although this may be ultimately less useful than that seen with CMR. The uptake of thallium (Tl-201) is an active process and requires intact myocardial cellular function, which implies viability. In particular late images after reinjection at 3–4 hours may show a degree of redistribution of Tl-201, which correlates with viability and/or hibernation. The value of even longer intervals of up to 24 hours is being investigated. Technetium-based sestamibi and tetrofosmin do not share these properties of thallium and are used less for this indication, although the addition of a nitrate injection is extending the role of technetium as a tracer in this cohort.

Day case angiography: patient selection

Most catheter labs routinely perform day case cardiac catheterization, and some are moving towards day case percutaneous intervention (PCI). This has significant advantages because it reduces expensive bed occupancy, and is often preferred by the patient. Therefore, this strategy needs to be achieved without increase in periprocedural risk to the patient. It is reasonable to assume suitability for a day case non-interventional procedure as the default strategy, providing that the following simple exclusions are observed in preprocedural checks and the periprocedural period. The presence of any of the following should trigger provisional planning to allow an overnight stay if it proves to be necessary:

- High risk due to left main disease, i.e. global ischaemia or hypotension on ETT, or marked peripheral vascular disease
- Heart failure
  - Pulmonary oedema
  - Severe/decompensated heart failure
- Ischaemia
  - Periprocedural ischaemia
  - Post-infarction ischaemia
- Severe valve disease
  - Severe aortic stenosis with LV dysfunction
  - Severe aortic regurgitation with a pulse pressure ≥80 mmHg
- Problematic supervision
  - Generalized debility or dementia
  - Lack of 24 hour supervision at home post procedure
- Renal failure
- Contrast reaction
- Need for continuous anticoagulation therapy
  - Mechanical MVR with AF
- Vascular complication
  - Difficult puncture, haematoma or false aneurysm.

Radiation safety

This subject is important and often dealt with in a limited fashion as part of a typical training scheme. Ultimately, however, only two people suffer: the careless operator and the patient with radiation dermatitis. Radiation protection is under statutory control, and a senior radiographer and doctor will have a statutory role in monitoring/auditing exposure.

Training centres in the UK are obliged to provide theoretical training in radiation protection in accordance with the Ionizing Radiation (Medical Exposure) Regulations 2000. Radiation protection courses should cover the theoretical aspects of the core syllabus that has been agreed by the Cardiology SAC of the Royal College of Physicians and British Institute of Radiology (BIR)and has been validated by the Radiation Protection Committee of the BIR.

Basic physics definitions

The measure of exposure is the roentgen (R), which is a unit of radiation exposure defined by the amount of ionization per unit mass of air due to X-rays or gamma-rays and its units are coulombs per kg (C/kg) – 1 R is 2.58×10^{-4} C kg^{-1} in SI units. The rad (radiation absorbed dose) is the amount of energy absorbed per unit mass of material and is described in terms of grays (Gy), in which 1 Gy = 100 rad or 1 J/kg.

The amount of energy absorbed for the same exposure varies depending on the type of radiation and the tissue. This is described as the rem, which is a rad multiplied by a correction factor. In cardiology, the correction factor for X-rays and gamma-rays is 1, so rem and rad are equal. The units for rems are expressed in terms of sieverts (Sv). By convention, radiation effects are described in mSv and there are 10 mSv per rem. Tissue differences may be important; for soft tissues 0.9 rad is absorbed for every 1 R of exposure, whereas for bones 4 rad is absorbed for 1 R of exposure.

It should be remembered that absorbed dose does not demonstrate the biological effects of radiation exposure. The equivalent dose is a measure of radiation absorption that reflects the ability of the particular radiation type to cause cellular damage and is expressed in terms of sieverts (Sv) [1]. The equivalent dose is simply the absorbed dose, in grays, multiplied by the weighting factor of the radiation:

$$\text{Equivalent dose (Sv)} = \text{absorbed dose (Gy)} \times \text{WR}$$

For X-rays this value is 1, therefore the equivalent dose is numerically equal to absorbed dose (Table 1.8).

Different tissues have different sensitivities to a certain equivalent dose of radiation and since the body is often not uniformly exposed to radiation, the concept of effective dose was developed. The effective

Table 1.8   Weighting factors for different radiation types

Type of radiation	Weighting factor of radiation
X-rays, γ-rays and electrons	1
Protons and thermal neutrons	5
Fast neutrons	5–20
A-particles and fission fragments	20

Table 1.9   Relative weighting factors for tissue or organ type

Tissue or organ	Weighting factor
Gonads	0.2
Red bone marrow	0.12
Lung	0.12
Stomach	0.12
Colon	0.12
Thyroid	0.05
Oesophagus	0.05
Liver	0.05
Bladder	0.05
Breast	0.05
Skin	0.01
Bone surfaces	0.01
Remainder	0.05
Total	1

dose is the sum of the equivalent doses to all tissues and organs of the body, multiplied by the weighting factor for each tissue or organ:

$$\text{Effective dose (Sv)} = +\text{ET} \times \text{WT}$$

where ET is the equivalent dose and WT is the weighting factor for a specific tissue or organ.

The International Commission on Radiological Protection (ICRP) provide figures for the weighting factors of the different tissues and organs (Table 1.9).

Previously, annual dose exposure has been set at 5 rem or 50 mSv, but increasingly there is a push to an annual dose limit of 2 rem or a lifetime exposure of 1 rem per year of life. More recently, the Ionizing Radiation Regulations (1999) provide guidelines on suitable levels of radiation exposure for medical staff in radiology and suggest that the effective dose should only be 20 mSv in any calendar year. In addition certain specifics are also suggested, as listed in Table 1.10.

Table 1.10   Maximum effective dose for specific tissue exposure

Area	Effective dose per year (mSv)
Lens of the eye	150
Skin	500
Hands, forearms, feet and ankles	500

Radiation protection training

The European Commission published specific guidelines for the accreditation of radiation protection training including specific learning objectives and 20–30 hours of training for interventional cardiologists [7].

The radiation dose received by staff, as recorded by personal dosimeters, includes the contribution of natural background radiation. The average background radiation dose to a person is 2.2 mSv every year. Background radiation exposure originates from three main natural sources: cosmic radiation, radiation from terrestrial sources and radioactivity within the body. The remaining sources of radiation are artificial and include, to a minute degree, radioactive waste and fallout from weapons testing. Inclusion of medically derived radiation, where diagnostic X-rays predominate, increases the average background radiation dose up to 2.6 mSv [8]. Although the average effective dose from these sources is very low in the general population, those in frequent contact with radiation occupationally can receive slightly more radiation dose. The average effective dose to an operator during each fluoroscopy-guided interventional procedure varies between 40 and 160 μSv. This dose correlates to completing between 125 and 500 interventional procedures each year for an individual cardiologist to reach the maximum legal annual limit. The mean effective dose actually received by most cardiologists falls far below this UK legal limit of 20 mSv. Indeed, any radiation worker whose radiation dose approaches or exceeds 6 mSv/year are at risk and therefore termed 'classified'. This term identifies those practitioners who have exceeded the recommended dose and are thus subject to more intense scrutiny of ongoing radiation exposure. In practical terms, few classified medical staff are present in the NHS.

There are two useful terms for describing the nature of radiation damage: stochastic and deterministic.

- *Stochastic risk* is where the severity of the resulting injury (i.e. gene damage or cancer) is the same, irrespective of dose, but the probability of developing the disease goes up. You do not develop a worse cancer because of a high radiation exposure compared with a low exposure, but you are much more likely to develop a gene defect or cancer with high dose rather than low dose.

- *Deterministic risk* is where the cumulative risk goes up with cumulative dose. For example cataract formation.

Since radiation carcinogenesis is a stochastic effect, the risk of cancer increases with the cumulative lifetime radiation dose increases. These effects usually present years after exposure to radiation. Radiation effective dose augments the baseline lifetime risk of fatal cancer by approximately 4 per cent Sv^{-1} $year^{-1}$ of absorbed dose [8]. For example, an interventional cardiologist who receives an effective dose of 1 mSv $year^{-1}$ and practises for 25 years will have a lifetime occupational exposure of 25 mSv. Thus the additional lifetime risk of cancer owing to radiation is 4 per cent $\times$ 0.025, or 0.1 per cent higher than the average risk.

Radiation measurement is achieved by one of two methods: either a film badge or a transluminescent dosimeter (TLD) badge. The film badge basically contains a piece of X-ray film, which is gradually fogged by X-rays. The exposure is roughly linearly proportional to the X-ray exposure. The TLD badge contains a disk with lithium fluoride crystals. The crystal absorbs the X-rays, and emit light in proportion to the degree of X-ray exposure.

If a single badge is worn, it is usually placed on the lead thyroid collar. Ideally, however, two badges should be worn, the second at the waist, underneath the lead apron, on the side from which the X-rays originate. This gives an estimation of exposure to the gonadal cells, which are perhaps the most radiation-sensitive cells in the body.

Radiation protection is based on three primary principles: time, distance and barriers, as well as minimizing exposure to scattered radiation. Obviously minimization of fluoroscopic and cine time results in a lower radiation exposure during cardiac catheterization. Similarly, since the intensity of the radiation beam is proportional to the inverse of the distance squared ($1/d^2$), the further from the source of scatter the operator is, the lower the radiation dose. The majority of scattered radiation at diagnostic energies is mainly backscatter, therefore if the tube is orientated under the table, then the majority of scattered radiation is directed at the floor. Inevitably there is variation in the type of X-ray equipment used in cardiac catheter laboratories, and older systems may have higher levels of radiation. More significant to the reduction of X-ray exposure is the employment of reasonable protective measures, including under-table guards and mobile ceiling-suspended shields, and the use of operator protection: lead apron, lead skirt, thyroid shield and potentially lead shin guards, helmet and glasses.

Radiation protection is a product of an interaction between the following:

- Imaging equipment and maintenance
- Radiation reduction strategies by radiographers
- Radiation reduction strategies by operators.

IMAGING EQUIPMENT AND MAINTENANCE

This is usually outside the remit of the trainee, but we will cover it briefly here. Part of the IR(ME)R regulations lay down statutory responsibilities of the employing organization to log all equipment in the unit using ionizing radiation. The requirements regarding the maintenance of equipment is less clear, but regular audit of dose levels is obligatory. When cumulative doses levels begin to rise, the organization contravenes its obligations to minimize X-ray exposure to patients and staff.

The employer needs to establish referral criteria for medical exposures, including an idea of relative radiation doses of those procedures. The resulting procedures will contribute to the cumulative radiation dose of individual patients and operators. Consequently the employer is obliged to set up a number of core operational procedures:

- To provide quality assurance programmes for standard procedures (i.e. setting appropriate monitoring and servicing of equipment).
- To define diagnostic reference levels for radiation-based examinations.
- To undertake continuing education and training, as part of IR(ME)R.
- To reporting of any accidental over- or unnecessary exposure.
- To audit whenever diagnostic reference levels are consistently exceeded, ensuring that corrective action is taken.

THE OBLIGATIONS OF THE DOCTOR

The IR(ME)R regulations specify certain roles, such as operator, practitioner and referrer:

- *Operator*: This is any person who is entitled to carry out the investigation, usually the cardiologist in our instance. However, it may also be scrub nurses if they depress the foot pedal under the direct supervision of a person who is adequately trained.

- *Practitioner*: This is the registered medical practitioner who takes responsibility for the exposure and is usually the consultant cardiologist whose patient it is or on whose list the procedure is being performed. The practitioner is responsible for the justification of a medical radiation exposure.
- *Referrer*: This means anyone who is entitled, in accordance with the employer's procedures, to refer individuals for medical X-ray exposure to a practitioner. This may include doctors and authorized nurses.

The referrer should give the practitioner sufficient information to enable a decision to be made as to whether the procedure is justified in terms or risk versus benefit:

- To consider the diagnostic or therapeutic benefits to the individual and the benefits to society. This allows the production of teaching material
- To assess the harm that the exposure may cause
- To consider available alternative techniques that have less exposure to ionizing radiation.

Obviously the consultant cardiologist may fulfil all three roles simultaneously: those of operator, practitioner and referrer. This is because they will make the clinical decision to investigate the patient with a test that involves radiation, justify the radiation exposure and carry out the procedure.

OPTIMIZATION

The key phrase in the radiation guidelines in the UK and the USA is to achieve a radiation dose as low as reasonably possible. This places the emphasis on the operator to select equipment and methods to ensure that for each medical exposure the dose of ionizing radiation to the individual undergoing the exposure is as low as possible. This can be achieved by:

- Institutional quality assurance
- Assessment of patient radiation dose

- Adherence to diagnostic reference levels set out in the employer's procedures
- Careful assessment of research projects involving radiation:
  - Patients'/subjects' participation must be voluntary
  - Individuals must know in advance about the risks of the exposure
  - Institutional dose constraints must be adhered to.

FLUOROSCOPY

When fluoroscopy is being used the operator is obliged to keep the dose as low as possible, which involves important co-operation with the radiographer, not only for the operator's own exposure but also for other members of the catheter lab staff who may be mobile within the lab. This can be achieved using the following guidelines:

- Keep screening times as low as possible
  - Less than 10 minutes for most procedures
  - Only use fluoroscopy when looking at the screen
- Spend less time acquiring images – the exposure is 10 times higher with acquisition mode than with screening mode
  - Only acquire images that contribute to the case
  - Keep acquisition runs short, but adequate for the required purpose.
- Cone down on the area of interest using the in-built shields in the X-ray equipment.
- Keep the image intensifier as close to the patient as possible
- Work in views that use less X-ray to penetrate or scatter (caudal views in general use more radiation than straight RAO or LAO views; similarly backscatter is greater from LAO or lateral than from AP)
- Use the lead screens provided, such as a lead skirt around the table and a mobile head/eye screen
- Treat your lead apron with respect
  - Hang it up, do not sling it on the back of a chair. If it develops a crack, it will be missed until the annual inspection, and you will have had additional exposure (Figure 1.2)
  - Make sure it is long enough
  - Always wear a thyroid guard
  - Consider shin guards

It is a salutary fact than only about 1 per cent of generated radiation actually is received by the image intensifier, and most is stopped by the

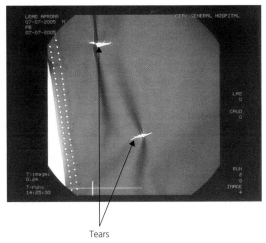

Tears

Figure 1.2   Protective X-ray apron with breaches through misuse.

patients skin. During a typical diagnostic procedure, the patient's dose can approach 50 R, or approximately 100–250 chest X-ray equivalents. As little as 200 R is needed to generate skin erythema. The primary operator will typically receive 1/1000 of the patient's dose, and the secondary operator/assistant 1/10 000 of the patient's dose as radiation dose reduces in proportion to the inverse square of the distance from the source.

The risk of radiation burns relates to prolonged procedures, where the C arm is not moved around and a single view is overly used. This is rare in diagnostic angiographic procedures, and is seen mostly in prolonged angioplasty or electrophysiology procedures. It can be minimized by changing views, and keeping screening and acquisition time to the minimum in prolonged procedures.

Image storage

The technical developments in medical imaging are rapid, with important improvements being made in the X-ray dose, quality of images and data storage. The X-rays are generated in a tube. This produces a lot of heat and in the past runs needed to be short to allow the tube to cool down between acquisitions. Modern tubes, however, have higher heat capacities so this is not so much of an issue. The X-ray beam exits the tube and passes towards the patients. Most will scatter back, causing locally increased exposure, but a small amount is passed through the patient and enters the image intensifier. Recent improvements in image intensifier design have given them better conversion factors, less distortion and better spatial resolution. A typical $512 \times 512 \times 8$ bit matrix can resolve down to 0.2–0.3 mm, but a newer, 1024 matrix will resolve down to 0.1–0.15 mm. The downside is that this has a significant impact on the size of file, and therefore on the hardware and software needed to archive and retrieve the files.

This process is almost entirely digital, which has generated the need for a universal standard. The Digital Imaging and Communications in Medicine (DICOM) is now established as the universal format, easily stored onto CD, DVD or hard disk. Increasingly we are moving towards more flexible desktop systems for viewing DICOM images for coronary angiographic procedures. However many files are very large, often many hundreds of megabytes in size, and many local IT networks cannot deal with these file sizes. Although there are a number of compression strategies available to make the files smaller as they are extracted from the archive and downloaded to the workstation, the American College of Cardiology/European Society of Cardiology (ACC/ESC) recommend that images used for clinical decision making should only be transported using lossless compression, typically 2:1. Files for non-clinical work can be transferred using higher compression strategies – lossy compression – which degrades the quality of the original image.

Patient preparation

The preparation of the patient is important, and can have severe consequences if not attended to conscientiously. It involves consideration of a complicated mix of factors, including:

- The identification of high-risk patients (diabetic, previous contrast reaction, chronic renal impairment, severe asthma, severe peripheral vascular disease, anticoagulation and valves)
- Baseline investigations
- Consent
- Premedication.

Preadmission checks

Initial outpatient assessment and/or preadmission clinics facilitate the identification and appropriate management of high-risk cases, reducing risk as far as practically possible for operator and patient alike. The preadmission clinic has a number of purposes:

- To ensure that high-risk patients are picked up and appropriate treatment pathways put in place (e.g. *N*-acetylcysteine in renal protection protocols)
- To ensure that important investigations such as ECGs, blood tests and even consent are gained in a quiet environment
- To provide a forum for patients to visit the lab, and ask questions
- To start clopidogrel prior to PCI.

It also needs to establish a minimum data set prior to safe angiography, including:

- Full blood count
- Urea and electrolytes (Na, K and creatinine)
- ECG
- Current medication list.

High risk patients

DIABETES

The diabetic patient covers a large spectrum of disease from the mildly insulin-resistant, diet-controlled patient, through to the patient with advanced brittle insulin-dependent diabetes. We tend to manage those using insulin together. They are type 1 patients (those with a failure of insulin production) and those whose insulin secretory capacity is no longer sufficient, despite the fact that they remain hyperinsulinaemic (the insulin-requiring type 2 diabetic). There are a number of factors that increase the risk for diabetic subjects:

- Prolonged procedures can induce hypoglycaemia
- Diabetes increases macrovascular disease
  - Difficulty with arterial access
  - Higher risk of left main stem and three vessel disease
  - Renal artery stenosis/renovascular disease

- Diabetes increases microvascular disease
  - Increased risk of renal medullary hypoxia and renal failure
  - Exacerbated with concurrent metformin prescription and contrast medium use
- Increased risk of access site complications (even when achieving arterial access has been straightforward).

When patients are listed for angiography, we identify concurrent diabetes and metformin use. This means that we can stop the metformin at least 48 hours in advance. Having said that, we have never seen a case of lactic acidosis when it has not been stopped in emergency situations. We also arrange the list order with knowledge of high-risk co-morbidities. This minimizes the chance, albeit low, of lactic acidosis when metformin, contrast-induced renal medullary hypoxia and patients with impaired renal function coincide. The recommendation is that it should be reintroduced 48 hours after the procedure.

Insulin-dependent/requiring patients
Our strategy for managing the insulin-dependent or requiring diabetic patient is as follows:

1. Arrange the diagnostic procedure first on the list to minimize risk of hypo- or hyperglycaemia. We try to utilize the morning list if possible, but the afternoon can be accommodated.
2. Allow a light, early breakfast ~6.00 am for morning procedures, with half dose insulin at the usual time.
3. Give normal breakfast and insulin if an afternoon procedure is contemplated, with a mid-morning snack 3 hours before the procedure.
4. Check blood glucose by BM stick pre and post procedure.
5. Allow the patient to eat and drink normally after the procedure and give a normal dose of insulin at tea time if adequate oral intake is achieved.
6. Only discharge the patient when eating and drinking.

Non-insulin-dependent patients
Diabetes is also a major cause of renal disease, and special attention needs to be paid to the renal function. Our strategy for managing the non-insulin-dependent diabetic patient is as follows:

1. Give light early breakfast.
2. Continue normal oral hypoglycaemic drug therapy – although metformin is withdrawn

3. Check blood glucose by BM stick pre and post procedure
4. Allow the patient to eat and drink normally after the procedure
5. Discharge the patient only if eating and drinking.

PREVIOUS CONTRAST REACTION

The previous occurrence of a contrast reaction is not a good predictor of future reactions. The relationship is even more uncertain if the previous reaction has been to intravenous agents, rather than intra-arterial injections. Although some undoubtedly have reproducible reactions to contrast agents, many do not. Even patients with previous catastrophic reactions to contrast may have an uneventful subsequent procedure.

Nevertheless, when faced with a patient who has had a previous contrast reaction, it is essential to take steps to minimize risk of adverse events. Appropriate strategies are as follows:

- Pretreat with prednisone 30 mg twice daily p.o. for 48 hours and chlorphenamine 10 mg three times daily for 48 hours.
- Undertake the procedure using isosmolar contrast medium using the minimum number of views.
- Give a test dose of 5 mL of contrast, and then wait for 3–5 minutes prior to carrying on with the rest of the test.
- Continue postprocedural treatment for a further 48 hours with both chlorphenamine and prednisone.

CHRONIC RENAL IMPAIRMENT

The coexistence of vascular disease and chronic renal failure is common. It presents a number of technical challenges to the cardiologist. Aorto-iliac disease is very common, creating problems accessing the heart from the femoral route. Figure 1.3 shows an angiographc image of a left iliac artery occlusion, after a failed right femoral puncture. There is a high incidence of hypertension, which may be severe, causing aortic root dilatation, making catheter selection more difficult. Finally, the presence of renovascular disease dramatically increases the incidence of contrast nephropathy. Adding diabetes to this volatile mix increases the risk of further deleterious effects on renal function.

Our protocol for dealing with patients with chronic renal impairment (creatinine >150 μmol/L) or patients who use continuous

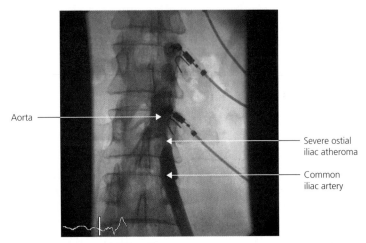

Aorta ——

—— Severe ostial
iliac atheroma

—— Common
iliac artery

Figure 1.3   Aorto-ostial iliac disease.

ambulatory peritoneal dialysis (CAPD) but who are not otherwise dialysis dependent, is as follows:

1. Identify the patient on the preadmission/booking sheet as having significant renal impairment and warranting renal impairment protocol.
2. Admit the patient the day prior to the procedure for at least 12 hours of prehydration and keep overnight for 12 hours postprocedural hydration. This is normally 1 L/12 hours of normal saline. Caution needs to be observed for those who are profoundly oligaemic but not yet dialysis dependent, as this can provoke pulmonary oedema.
3. Administer N-acetylcysteine for 48 hours pre and post procedure (600 mg p.o. twice daily), although evidence of efficacy remains debatable.
4. Undertake the procedure using the lowest number of views to allow a diagnostic decision to be made, to keep the burden of contrast as low as possible. We do not perform left ventricular angiography since this information can be obtained by non-invasive investigations such as echocardiography.
5. Use isotonic and isosmolar contrast medium to reduce the renal medullary insult. The downside is the increased viscosity as molecular size increases to reduce osmolarity, making these agents difficult to inject unless kept in the warmer until the last possible minute.

6. Avoid follow-on interventional procedures to minimize the additional contrast load, and schedule this for a later date. It may take some weeks for the renal function to return to baseline, if it does at all.
7. Make arrangements to check renal function either by an early outpatient appointment or through liaising with the general practitioner. The decline in renal function may peak on day 3–5 and may persist for several weeks.

Dialysis-dependent patients, excluding those who use CAPD as their renal replacement therapy, are often easier to manage. The critical point is the link with the dialysis unit, to ensure adequate renal replacement therapy soon after the procedure; whether this is CAPD, haemodialysis or haemofiltration.

The concern with this subset of patients is the fluid volume given during the procedure, as the patient has no way of removing this. It may be better to admit this group of patients after the procedure, with renal replacement therapy being instituted promptly after the procedure once haemostasis has been achieved, to prevent such difficulties arising. Obviously in this group N-acetylcysteine has little role to play.

The relationship with the nephrologists cannot be overemphasized. Their patients have a lot of heart disease and our patients have a lot of renal disease. It is well worth fostering close links with the renal unit.

SEVERE PERIPHERAL VASCULAR DISEASE

This group of patients can also be very difficult to manage. However, with access through bilateral radial and femoral arteries described later in this book, most patients can undergo angiography. Problems with puncturing through femoral grafts are discussed in Chapter 4.

ANTICOAGULATION AND VALVES

Patients may be taking anticoagulants for a number of reasons as listed in Table 1.11.

Patients with mechanical valves present particular problems to the cardiologist, because there are incumbent risks attached to the withdrawal of anticoagulation. Running the INR down to between 1.5 and 1.8 to facilitate femoral puncture is reasonable in patients with aortic mechanical valve replacements, because the high velocity flow through

Table 1.11   Indications for anticoagulation and intravenous antiplatelet agents

Anticoagulants	Possible indications
Warfarin/coumadin	Mechanical valves
	Atrial fibrillation
	Thromboembolic syndromes such as deep vein thrombosis or pulmonary embolism
	Left ventricular thrombus
Heparin	Post acute coronary syndromes
Glycoprotein IIb–IIIa inhibitors	Post acute coronary syndromes

the valve reduces the risk of clot deposition on the valve. Below 1.5 INR heparin needs to be started.

Mechanical mitral valves are at much higher risk of thrombus deposition and particular care must be taken. The femoral operator has to withdraw warfarin to achieve an INR <1.8 and start heparin to maintain anticoagulation. We would normally stop heparin 4 hours prior to the case starting. We would pull the sheath afterwards and restart heparin after 2 hours. We would then reload with warfarin to achieve INR >2.0. Needless to say, this patient should be admitted to hospital.

The use of femoral closure devices is increasingly common, but expensive. We reserve them for those patients catheterized via the femoral route, whose INR is >2.0. Routine use is expensive, and femoral complications including false aneurysm still occur. These devices are discussed later in Chapter 4.

Radial operators can run a normal therapeutic INR between 2 and 3, ignore the additional heparin given during radial procedures and discharge the patient home on their normal dose of warfarin. Therefore the radial approach offers significant advantages in this population. The technique of radial artery cardiac catheterization and right heart catheterization from the antecubital vein in an anticoagulated patient is discussed in Chapter 3.

Vitamin K

We try to avoid using vitamin K, because it makes the re-anticoagulation of the patient difficult for some days and occasionally weeks. In the patient with a femoral angiogram, a mechanical mitral valve and atrial fibrillation the use of vitamin K can commit the patient to anticoagulation with intravenous heparin for a long period of time. Prolonged exposure to unfractionated heparin increases the likelihood of developing heparin-induced

Table 1.12   Major complication of cardiac catheterization

Complication	Percentage risk	Incidence
Risk of death	0.08%	1:1250
Risk of myocardial infarction	0.03%	1:3333
Risk of neurological injury	0.06%	1:1600
Major vascular complication	0.4%	1:250

thrombocytopenia syndrome (HITS). As yet temporary anticoagulation with low molecular weight heparin cannot be recommended.

The risks of basic cardiac catheter lab investigations

Each institution should be able to generate their own institutional risk assessment for major and minor complications, especially as national catheter lab data sets are now collected in almost all catheter laboratories.

The 1990 data from the SCA&I on the percentage risks for a diagnostic cardiac catheter are shown in Table 1.12.

Admission procedure

The patient should be admitted by the nurses, to ensure the basics such as the preadmission data set is complete and available.

Intravenous access

Ideally, this should be secured in all patients. However, in many units the majority of day-case procedures are very low risk and intravenous access is not secured routinely. Nevertheless, complications such as anaphylaxis, contrast reaction and ischaemia can be unexpected, rapid and progressive even in seemingly low-risk diagnostic procedures. The extra time it takes to obtain venous access can be critical in an emergency. A 21G cannula should be in the antecubital vein or a proximal forearm vein for all cases as a small-gauge intravenous cannula in the back of the hand is almost useless when fluid replacement needs to be given rapidly. If this is not routine in the lab, then any suspicion of increased risk such as diabetes, evidence of peripheral vascular disease, previous drug reactions or clinical instability should mandate intravenous access being a prerequisite for the catheterization.

> **Critical safety point**: A 21G cannula should be in the antecubital vein or a proximal forearm vein for all at-risk cases.

Sedation

The use of sedation is at the discretion of the operator, bearing in mind the needs of the patient. We do not routinely give sedation for our investigative or therapeutic procedures, unless excessive anxiety is reported.

Intravenous sedation requires conscious sedation protocols to be followed, including the need for supplemental oxygen during the procedure, as well as oxygen saturation monitoring by pulse oximetry. We recommend the administration of a small dose of a short-acting anxiolytic such as midazolam, titrated against clinical response. Although, oral sedation as a premedication warrants no further monitoring during the procedure its efficacy is varied and unpredictable and we do not recommend it.

Allen's test

We run a large radial programme in Stoke, although there are still some steadfast femoral operators. Our catheter lab nurses have become very adept at performing Allen's test. However, there are now data to suggest that this test of dual blood supply of the hand does not predict radial access site complications. A number of high-profile European cardiac units have abandoned it as a screening procedure. As yet, we have not gone this far. We do have a low threshold for assessing radial and ulnar arterial flow by Doppler, but even this does not provide a good assessment of hand blood flow. It is discussed in Chapter 3.

Preprocedural ECG

This should be standard in all patients undergoing intervention and EP, but not necessarily all diagnostic angiography.

Consent

The issue of consent is an important one, although one often skipped over for speed or in an attempt not to scare a very anxious patient. However it can cause medicolegal problems when complications (do!) arise. A number of issues have been resolved by institutions driving the reform of the consent process, but the individual doctor's attitude to consent remains crucial.

Consent is required every time a procedure is undertaken, and is regarded as a process rather than a single event. Consent can be written, verbal or implied. However, when the situations allow it, written consent is perhaps easier to defend. The General Medical Council in the UK makes it clear that the doctor who is undertaking treatment or investigation should be responsible for ensuring that the patient has given consent prior to the event. It suggests that the practitioner should be capable of carrying out the procedure, or be able to demonstrate training has been given in order to be able to gain consent.

Withdrawal of consent or refusal of treatment

There are a number of very difficult situations regarding consent. The withdrawal of consent is one of them. Any competent person may withdraw consent for a procedure/investigation at any time.

A competent patient may refuse treatment or investigation even if the potential consequences are dire. Examples such as Jehovah's Witnesses refusing blood products, even if failure to do may cause death, are well known. Competence to make rational decisions is assumed for any adult over the age of 16 years, unless there is convincing evidence to the contrary. However, a decision with which the doctor profoundly disagrees and regards as illogical, irrational or unjustified is not, in itself, evidence of incompetence. The patient should be able to:

- Understand in simple language what medical treatment is being proposed
- Understand its benefits, risks and alternatives
- Understand in broad terms the consequences of not receiving the proposed treatment
- Retain and assess the information in order to arrive at a balanced decision.

The extent of information

There is a gradual move towards a more North American model of extensive consent forms, in the hope of preventing litigation. However, the main thrust of consent is not to apportion blame for a perhaps rare and unfortunate complication of a procedure, but rather to provide the majority of lay people with enough information to make an informed choice about a particular investigation or treatment pathway. The essence of the GMC guidance on the type of information doctors should provide is as follows.

- The purpose of the investigation or treatment
- Options for treatment, which should include the option not to treat
- Explanation of the likely benefits, likelihood of success and possible side effects
- The name of the supervising doctor
- A reminder that the patient can change his or her mind at any time.

Advance statements and directives

Advance statements (or living wills) can take a number of forms, and can govern the way we act as doctors even when faced with a patient who is clearly no longer competent to make his or her own decision regarding investigation and treatment. It may take the form of a written statement or it can be a verbal statement, although this presents obvious difficulties to the doctor who may be faced with a ill patient and an unknown relative, suggesting no treatment be undertaken. An even worse predicament can occur where conflicting opinions are offered from elements within the same family. Some advance statements suggest another adult who has been identified to make those difficult decisions.

A clear, written statement refusing particular medical interventions (usually termed an advance directive) should be regarded as binding on the doctor.

Further reading

Office of Public Sector. Statutory Instrument 1999 no. 32. *The Ionizing Radiations Regulations 1999*. www.opsi.gov.uk/si/si1999/19993232.htm

Bashore TM *et al*. Cardiac Catheterization Laboratory Standards: a report of the American College of Cardiology Task Force on Clinical Expert Consensus Documents (ACC/SCA&I Committee to Develop an Expert Consensus Document on Cardiac Catheterization Laboratory Standards). *J Am Coll Cardiol* 2001; **37:** 2170–2214.

General Medical Council. *Seeking Patients' Consent: the Ethical Considerations.* November 1998. http://www.gmc-uk.org/guidance/library/consent.asp

References

1. Bashore TM, Bates ER, Berger PB *et al.* American College of Cardiology/Society for Cardiac Angiography and Interventions Clinical Expert Consensus Document on cardiac catheterization laboratory standards. A report of the American College of Cardiology Task Force on Clinical Expert Consensus Documents. *J Am Coll Cardiol* 2001; **37:** 2170–2214.
2. British Cardiac Society and the Specialty Advisory Committee in Cardiovascular Medicine of the Royal College of Physicians. *Guidelines for Specialist Training in Cardiology,* 2002.
3. Johnson LW and Krone R. Cardiac catheterization 1991: a report of the Registry of the Society for Cardiac Angiography and Interventions (SCA&I). *Cathet Cardiovasc Diag* 1993; **28:** 219–220.
4. Johnson LW, Lozner EC, Johnson S *et al.* Coronary arteriography 1984–1987: a report of the Registry of the Society for Cardiac Angiography and Interventions. I. Results and complications. *Cathet Cardiovasc Diag* 1989; **17:** 5–10.
5. ACC/AHA Committee. ACC/AHA 2002 guideline update for exercise testing: summary article: A report of the American College of Cardiology/American Heart Association task force on practice guidelines (Committee to Update the 1997 Exercise Testing Guidelines). *J Am Coll Cardiol* 2002; **40:** 1531–1540.
6. Gianrossi R, Detrano R, Mulvihill D *et al.* Exercise-induced ST depression in the diagnosis of coronary artery disease. A meta-analysis. *Circulation* 1989; **80:** 87–98.
7. Vano E. Radiation exposure to cardiologists: how it could be reduced. *Heart (British Cardiac Society).* 2003; **89:** 1123–1124.
8. National Radiological Protection Board. *Living with Radiation,* 5th edn. Chilton: NRPB, 1998.

Coronary anatomy, physiology and pharmacology

2

The anatomy of coronary artery and veins

Left coronary anatomy

The left coronary artery (LCA) arises from the left coronary sinus of Valsalva of the aortic root in the vast majority of cases, and is the first of the aortic branches. It can arise both from the non-coronary (posterior) and right coronary sinus, but this is unusual. Typically it will arise from within the upper third of the sinus, but can occur higher up, up to the level of the sinotubular junction. Occasionally it may arise near a valve commissure. This can make engagement with a catheter technically demanding, because the ostium of the main stem, where it opens into the aorta, is obliquely orientated.

The LCA begins as the left main stem (LMS) and divides into its major branches – the left anterior descending (LAD), circumflex (Cx) and sometimes the intermediate (Int) arteries, which may be seen in approximately 30 per cent of cases. The LAD supplies blood to the anterior wall and anterior half of the septum. The Cx supplies the lateral wall and, if dominant, will supply the posterior wall and posterior portion of the septum. The right coronary artery (RCA) is dominant in about 85 per cent of cases and then supplies right ventricle (RV), posterior left ventricle (LV) wall and posterior septum.

The LMS is of variable length, although usually less than 10 mm long. It may occasionally be absent, with the LAD and Cx having separate origins arising from the left coronary sinus. Occasionally the origins of Cx and LAD just touch, which is usually termed conjoint. However, separate or conjoint origins are uncommon and account for less than 1 per cent of cases. The main stem usually passes between the right hand margin of the left atrial appendage and left hand border of the main pulmonary artery (MPA). The major branches – LAD and Cx – both then take predominantly subendocardial courses, as the former runs in the interventricular groove and the latter in the atrioventricular (AV) groove (Figure 2.1).

The LAD usually gives off a major first diagonal branch that passes posteriorly and supplies the anterior free wall of the heart. The LAD also gives off a variable number of arteries perpendicular to itself, to pass into the muscular septum. The first septal artery usually arises within the first 10 mm of the LMS bifurcation, and is often an obvious and sizeable vessel, whereas those that emerge more distally are usually more numerous and much smaller. The subendocardial course of the LAD may be interrupted by segments where the artery passes intra-myocardially. These segments appear at angiography to be muscle bridging and present difficulties to the surgeon, who may then have problems in pacing graft conduit. In most cases, the LAD terminates after it has passed around the apex of the heart.

The Cx runs initially across the anterior superior margin of the left atrial appendage, before dropping into the AV groove, forming an arcade, with interconnections occasionally seen with the distal RCA. It gives off branches both posterosuperiorly to supply the left atrium and also inferoanteriorly to supply the obtuse marginal or lateral surface of the heart via the obtuse marginal (OM) vessels. Figure 2.2 shows a left dominant coronary system in an left anterior oblique (LAO) caudal view where the AV groove Cx comes all the way round to reach the posterior

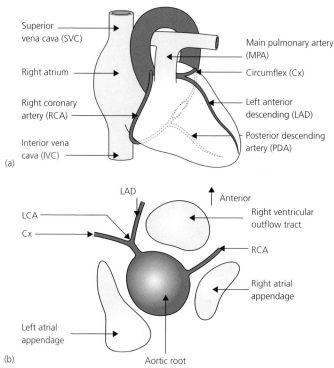

Figure 2.1 Origin and course of native coronary arteries.

interventricular groove. Figure 2.3 shows an LAO cranial view of a non-dominant LCA. Here the Cx terminates on the lateral surface and fails to come round to reach the posterior interventricular groove and therefore line up with the LAD.

Right coronary artery

The RCA normally arises in the right coronary sinus, but may also arise superiorly near the sinotubular junction or near the commissures. These slight anatomical variations can cause an enormous amount of trouble when trying to selectively intubate the ostium of the RCA. Engaging the LMS is usually straightforward, and preshaped catheters make this very easy. However, the RCA demands a degree of skill and dexterity even if it arises in its normal position. Similarly, whereas the LCA typically emerges as a single vessel, the RCA often has a number of small vessels

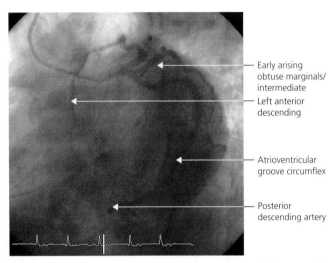

Early arising
obtuse marginals/
intermediate

Left anterior
descending

Atrioventricular
groove circumflex

Posterior
descending artery

Figure 2.2   Dominant left coronary artery (left anterior oblique caudal view).

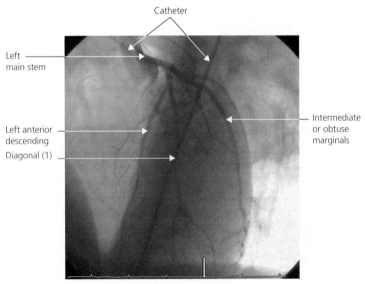

Catheter

Left
main stem

Left anterior
descending

Diagonal (1)

Intermediate
or obtuse
marginals

Figure 2.3   Left coronary artery with non-dominant circulation (left anterior oblique cranial view).

arising directly from the aorta which may supply sinus node or proximal pulmonary artery.

The proximal RCA drops away from the aortic root, posterior to the pulmonary artery, before entering the AV groove. It will usually give branches anteroinferiorly that supply the right ventricle, termed acute marginal vessels, and posterosuperiorly that supply the right atrium. Typically, the RCA gives off the posterior descending (PD) artery, as it crosses the intersection of AV groove and the interventricular groove, although this branch may arise more proximally and traverse across the inferior surface of the RV. The PD artery runs perpendicularly towards the left ventricular apex, in the interventricular groove, where it may form an arcade with the LAD. The PD artery gives off perpendicular branches superiorly to supply the inferior septum. The RCA continues as the crux artery, giving a branch to the AV node and then branches to the posterolateral surface of the heart via the posterior lateral (PL) arteries. In approximately 80 per cent of cases the PD and PL arteries arise from the RCA. In 10 per cent of cases, they arise from the Cx, and the LCA is referred to as dominant. In the last remaining 10 per cent, the circulation is said to be balanced, when these arteries arise from both Cx and RCA. Figure 2.4 shows a non-dominant RCA seen in right anterior

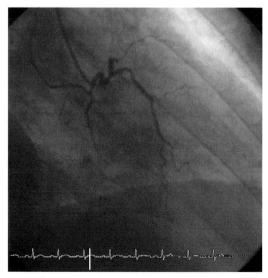

Figure 2.4   Non-dominant right coronary artery (right anterior oblique view).

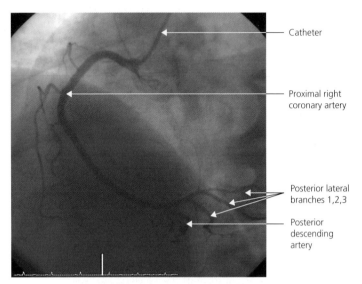

Catheter

Proximal right coronary artery

Posterior lateral branches 1,2,3

Posterior descending artery

Figure 2.5 Right coronary artery with dominant circulation (anteroposterior cranial view).

oblique view. There is no significant vessel in the AV groove, and only the RV and right atrium (RA) are supplied. Figure 2.5 shows a dominant RCA in anteroposterior (AP) cranial view. This is often a very good view for opening out the RCA/PD artery bifurcation.

Normal coronary vein anatomy

There are two major groups of veins in the heart (Figure 2.6): those that drain into the coronary sinus and those that drain directly into the cardiac chambers – the Thesbian and anterior cardiac veins. The anterior cardiac veins drain blood from the anterior aspect of the heart directly into the right atrium.

There are three main tributaries of the coronary sinus: the great, middle and small cardiac veins. The entrance to the sinus is guarded by the crescent-shaped Thesbian valve.

- *Great cardiac vein*: This vessel follows the initial course of the LAD in the anterior interventricular groove, thereby draining the anterior wall and anterior septum, before entering the left AV groove alongside the circumflex. It picks up the venous drainage of the OM vessels on the lateral surface. It terminates in the coronary sinus.

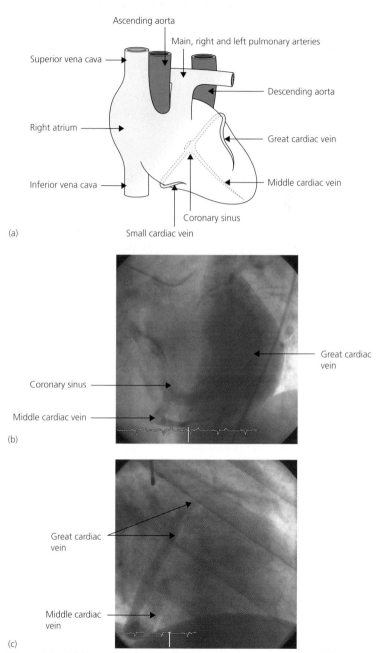

Figure 2.6 (a) Venous drainage of the heart, (b) in left anterior oblique cranial and (c) right anterior oblique views.

- *Middle cardiac vein*: This vessel follows the PD artery in the posterior interventricular groove, and drains the inferior wall and posterior septum.
- *Small cardiac vein*: This traverses the RV free wall, with the marginal branches of the RCA, before entering the AV groove and terminating in the coronary sinus.

Anatomy of heart and great vessels

The anatomical information about the heart that can be obtained from cardiac catheterization is relatively limited. Certainly echocardiography, computerized tomography (CT) and magnetic resonance imaging (MRI) offer far greater structural anatomical information. However, angiography can provide important information regarding pressure gradients across valves, directly across the aortic, tricuspid and pulmonary and indirectly across the mitral valve. It can also provide important information regarding aortic and mitral regurgitation and LV function.

Venous inflow

There are two main caval veins: the superior vena cava (SVC), which drains head, neck, thorax and upper limbs, and the inferior vena cava (IVC), which drains the remainder.

SUPERIOR VENA CAVA

The axillary vein turns into the subclavian at the inferolateral border of the first rib. Each brachiocephalic vein is in turn generated by the insertion of the internal jugular veins into the subclavian vein, which has already received the external jugular vein. The SVC is made from the confluence of the right and left brachiocephalic veins (also termed the innominates), the left being longer than the right. The SVC inserts into the right atrium, after receiving the azygos vein that drains the thorax. The venous system sits anatomically in front of the corresponding arterial vessels.

INFERIOR VENA CAVA

The IVC returns all blood from below the diaphragm. It is formed from the confluence of the iliac veins as they emerge from the pelvis. It continues anterior to the spine and to the right of the aorta. It receives the two renal veins, the two suprarenal veins and the hepatic and phrenic veins.

This anatomy is only important when accessing the heart from the femoral veins, when the catheter can (and does regularly) enter every branch. For example, when having to insert an emergency temporary pacing wire from the femoral route, entering the phrenic veins can explain the pacing wire appearing to be in the right place, but no RV capture can be achieved.

Right atrium

The RA has a number of structures that drain into it. However, the angiographic appearance is rarely studied. The posterior portion of the right atrium converges into the tricuspid valve. Figure 2.7 shows a right atrial angiogram which is followed through the RV and pulmonary artery with a long acquisition run. The IVC and SVC are not seen in this view.

Tricuspid valve

As its name suggests, the tricuspid valve has three leaflets: septal, anterosuperior and inferior. The junction of each leaflet is termed a

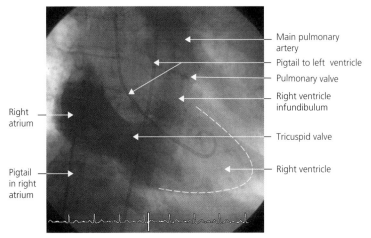

Figure 2.7 Right atrial and right ventriculogram (right anterior oblique view).

commissure, and each is support by chordae tendinae, fibrous cords that arise from the papillary muscles and insert into the valve leaflets. The anteroseptal commissure, the junction between septal and antero-superior leaflets, is supported by the medial papillary muscle. The anteroinferior commissure is supported by the anterior papillary muscle. There is no specific inferior papillary muscle. There is no fibrous annulus to support the tricuspid valve, which is why it is prone to functional dilatation in right heart disease. Instead it is supported by an infolding of the AV groove and therefore lies in close proximity to the RCA.

Right ventricle

The RV has a banana-shaped cavity in transverse section but is more triangular in shape when considered in a coronal section, which wraps around the more conical LV. This complex three-dimensional shape is also the reason why right ventriculography is not commonly used, as the results obtained are visually difficult to interpret. The inflow comes from the tricuspid valve on the right side of the cavity, with the papillary muscles and chordae tendinae orientated towards the RV apex. Above this is the RV outflow tract or infundibulum, which is a muscular tube which provides support for the pulmonary valve.

Pulmonary valve

The pulmonary valve has three leaflets. Two face the aorta, which sits directly behind the aortic valve. These have been termed the right- and left-facing leaflets, the third being termed the non-facing leaflet. This orientation cannot be appreciated at catheterization.

Pulmonary arteries

The main pulmonary artery begins above the infundibulum of the RV and the pulmonary valve. It is located anteriorly to the aorta, and passes posteriorly, before it divides into the two main branches, the right and left pulmonary arteries, and enters the hilum of the respective lung. The right pulmonary artery (RPA) takes a right angle, passing horizontally into the right lung, and is best seen in the posteroanterior view. The left pulmonary artery (LPA) is slightly longer and proceeds almost directly posteriorly, passing over the left main bronchus. Each pulmonary artery

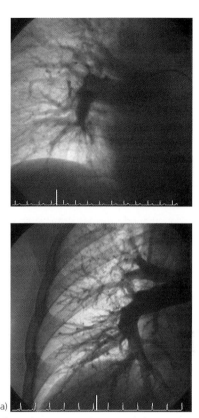

Figure 2.8 (a) Right pulmonary angiogram: right anterior oblique (top) and posteroanterior (bottom) views.

then subdivides to supply the bronchopulmonary segments of each lung. The LPA is best seen in the LAO 45° view. It is worth noting that there is huge individual variation (Figure 2.8).

The LPA divides into eight major branches: four supply the upper lobe (including two to the lingula) and four supply the lower lobe. These typically emerge as two short trunks supplying upper and lower lobes, which then subdivide into the four branches to each lobe.

The RPA divides into three short trunks, which then subdivide again: three to the anterior lobe, two to the middle lobe and five to the inferior lobe.

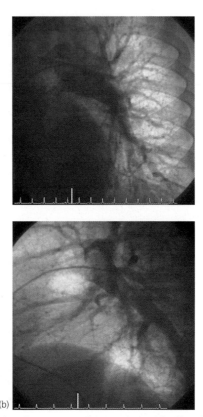

Figure 2.8   (b) Left pulmonary angiogram: lateral (top) and left anterior oblique (bottom) views.

Left atrium

This chamber is the most posterior, and is anatomically best seen either by transoesophageal echocardiography (TOE) or by gated cardiac magnetic resonance (CMR). It is rarely directly visualized by angiography, unless a right ventriculogram has been performed, and the operator waits for the passage of contrast through the lungs for a second phase angiogram of the left atrium (LA). The presence of an atrial septal defect (ASD) would allow direct injection through the defect, but TOE and CMR are still the imaging investigations of choice.

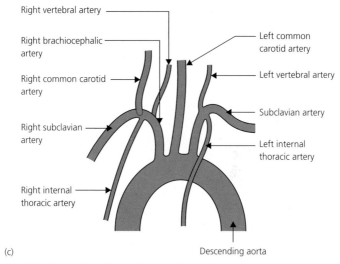

Right vertebral artery

Right brachiocephalic artery

Right common carotid artery

Right subclavian artery

Right internal thoracic artery

Left common carotid artery

Left vertebral artery

Subclavian artery

Left internal thoracic artery

(c)

Descending aorta

Figure 2.8 (c) Aortic arch and the great vessels.

The chamber is bounded posteriorly by a smooth-walled venous component, which receives the four pulmonary veins that drain oxygenated blood from the lung into the LA. Anteriorly is the trabeculated LA appendage. It is smaller and the transition from LA to LA appendage less well defined than with the RA and RA appendage. Inferiorly it is bound by the mitral valve.

Mitral valve

This valve has two leaflets, although terminologies can make this confusing. Cardiologists will normally discuss the mitral valve in terms of having an anterior and posterior leaflet. Some anatomists will discuss the valve as having aortic and mural leaflets, representing anterior and posterior respectively.

The anterior leaflet is tongue shaped, with the line of closure with the posterior leaflet being almost a semi-circle. The valve is supported inferiorly by the anterior papillary muscle and accompanying chordae for its anterior half and the posterior papillary muscle and chordae for its posterior half. The anterior mitral valve (MV) leaflet is continuous with the aortic valve.

The posterior MV leaflet is crescent shaped, with three distinct scalloped segments. These are termed posterior 1–3 or P1, P2 and P3, with P1 being the most anterior. P1 is mainly supported by the anterior papillary muscle, and P3 by the posterior. P2 is supported by both. The number of scallops is variable, with between two and five being seen on otherwise healthy valves.

It is important to note that for efficient closure and haemodynamic competence the corresponding sections of anterior and posterior MV leaflets are supported by the same papillary muscle and chordae.

Left ventricle

This cavity generates systemic pressures and is the most muscular in the heart. Blood enters from the left atrium, through the MV, and is discharged through the aortic valve. It is muscular from mitral ring to the apex, and only a small portion of the superior interventricular septum is membranous.

The LV is extensively studied at angiography to assess LV function and to interrogate for the presence of septal defects. The LV appearance at angiography is described below in terms of segments and grades of movement in the two traditional views: RAO 30–40° and LAO 40–50°.

Aortic valve

The aortic valve is similar in anatomy to the pulmonary valve. It consists of three semilunar valves attached in the main to the fibrous trunk of the aorta and the upper muscular part of the septum, in three sinuses. The sinuses and valve leaflets are orientated so that two are pointed anteriorly and one posteriorly. They are usually named according to the coronary vessel that arises from the sinus: left (left anterior) and right (right anterior) coronary sinuses and the non-coronary (posterior) sinus.

Aortic arch

The aorta leaves the heart and initially forms the ascending aorta. It then typically gives three major branches: the right brachiocephalic trunk, the left common carotid and the left subclavian arteries

(Figure 2.8c). The right brachiocephalic trunk becomes the right sub-clavian after giving off the right common carotid artery.

Coronary artery nomenclature

The coronary systems have been labelled differently over the years, but the following represents the system seen in use most often in the UK.

Left main (LM)

By convention, this is the LCA before it bifurcates into LAD and Cx. If the RCA is very dominant and therefore the Cx very small, the LMS may in effect become an LAD as the anterior free wall and some of the obtuse marginal surface may only be supplied by diagonals. In this case it remains the LSM until the first branch.

Left anterior descending artery (LAD)

This vessel starts after the origin of the Cx and follows the interventric-ular septum round to the apex. It occasionally occurs as a double sys-tem (see below), giving two sets of branches: diagonals and septals.

DIAGONAL ARTERIES (D_{1-x})

Diagonal arteries are numbered sequentially beginning with the first vessel after the origin of the circumflex. They supply the anterior free wall. The first diagonal (D_1) usually arises before the first septal. In the LAO cranial view, the diagonals go to the right of the screen, whereas the septals go to the left as viewed by the operator.

SEPTAL ARTERIES (S_{1-x})

Septal arteries are also numbered sequentially, starting with the first vessel which enters the proximal portion of the septum after the origin of the LAD. Occasionally a septal may come off a large diagonal. If this occurs, the sequential numbering should be maintained.

Circumflex artery (Cx)

The Cx starts at the left main stem bifurcation, and runs in the AV groove. It gives a number of posteriorly directed branches towards the left atrium, the first of which may supply the sinus node.

Often in a right dominant system (about 80 per cent of the population), the larger vessel breaks out of the AV groove and crosses onto the lateral surface of the heart, becoming the obtuse marginal (OM) arteries. The AV groove is appreciated on moving RAO images as a slightly paler radiolucent area of pericardial fat in the AV groove. The Cx may continue as a much smaller vessel, often termed the AV circumflex artery. The OM vessels are labelled sequentially from the LM bifurcation. The intermediate artery is a cause of some confusion, and refers to an artery which arises from the LM, between LAD and Cx, creating a trifurcation. The additional branch should really be called OM_1, but is usually termed the intermediate (Int) artery, with the next OM being OM_2.

In a left dominant system (about 20 per cent of population), the larger vessel continues in the AV groove, until it approaches the junction of AV groove and posterior interventricular groove. At this juncture, it may give off the AV nodal artery posteriorly, before entering the interventricular groove as the PD artery (see Figure 2.2, page 40).

Right coronary artery (RCA)

The RCA enters the AV groove early, but prior to doing so, gives off the conus branch, which supplies the pulmonary infundibulum. The conus is more anteriorly directed, and supplies a tunnel of myocardium separating the aortic and pulmonary valves from the mitral and tricuspid valves. The second branch is usually a posteriorly directed branch to the sinus node. There are a variable number of right atrial branches that pass posteriorly and right ventricular branches that pass anteriorly, a distinction best seen in RAO view, where RV branches will be directed to the right of the screen as viewed by the operator and RA branches to the left. The RCA continues until it nears the junction of AV groove and posterior interventricular groove. At this juncture it divides into the crux artery, which continues in the AV groove and the PD artery, which enters the interventricular groove. The crux artery then will give off the AV nodal artery towards the atria and a number of posterolateral branches (PLBs), which supply the lateral wall. These are numbered sequentially after the PD artery as $PLB_{(1-x)}$.

Physiology

Coronary artery physiology

The role of the coronary arteries is to deliver sufficient blood to the myocardium at all levels of effort, a difficult task given that the heart has a high basal O_2 demand, 8–10 mL O_2/min/100 g, which may increase 10-fold during severe effort. This is the highest rate of extraction of O_2 of any organ. Of major importance is the fact that coronary flow is principally a diastolic phenomenon, particularly in the LAD and Cx territories, where the myocardial muscle mass can exert a high external compressive pressure, preventing systolic flow. When supplying the RV, the RCA is able to overcome the compressive force of RV contraction, allowing biphasic flow (i.e. flow in both systole and diastole). This reversal of the normal flow pattern renders the endocardial (internal) surface of the heart particularly susceptible to ischaemia.

Flow is governed by resistance vessels, which are not seen at angiography, although myocardial blush probably represents resistance arteriolar and capillary flow.

Overall vascular tone is the summation of local regulatory mechanisms and extrinsic influences in the coronary bed. The heart autoregulates its own blood flow very effectively between 60 and 200 mmHg.

A local regulatory mechanism is one that, by definition, can be demonstrated in an *in vitro* model to be separate from systemic control and to include local vasodilators such as nitric oxide, adenosine, prostaglandins and local hypoxia. Vasoconstrictors include agents such as endothelin, that contributes to homeostatic control. In the myogenic reflex, when an artery is suddenly dilated by a surge in pressure, endothelin acts locally to constrict it.

Extrinsic pathways include the sympathetic and parasympathetic nervous systems.

- *Sympathetic activation*: This initially causes a transient vasoconstriction via the direct effects of neuronally derived norepinephrine on the α_1 receptor, however this is rapidly overshadowed by the vasodilatation caused by β_1 receptor effects of norepinephrine, associated with increased force of contraction. Circulating adrenal-derived epinephrine predominantly affects cardiac β_2 adrenoreceptors, influencing vasodilatation. Norepinephrine and epinephrine are the recommended international names for noradrenaline and adrenaline, respectively.

- *Parasympathetic effects*: Parasympathetic activation causes modest vasodilatation due to a direct effect of acetylcholine on muscarinic (M_2) receptors, which then release nitric oxide. Autoregulation may be activated, however, if the heart rate falls dramatically and local mechanisms increase coronary resistance.

Physiology and cardiac output

Cardiac output (CO) is the product of heart rate (HR) and stroke volume (SV):

$$CO = HR \times SV$$

HEART RATE

HR is relatively easily understood and is under endocrine and neuro-endocrinal control. Heart rate can be increased and decreased. If SV is fixed, as is often the case in severe heart failure, an increase in heart rate may be the only way of increasing CO (Table 2.1).

STROKE VOLUME

Stroke volume is a more complicated topic than heart rate and only the bare bones will be presented here. The heart fills by a combination of passive and active mechanisms, and actively contracts to empty. This

Table 2.1 Physiological factors affecting heart rate

Factors	Causes
Factors that decrease heart rate	
Reduced sympathetic drive	Beta-blockers, cardiogenic syncope
Reduced epinephrine secretion	Adrenal failure
Increased parasympathetic drive	Cardiogenic syncope, muscarinic drugs
Factors that increase heart rate	
Increased sympathetic drive	Fight/flight response, stress, low cardiac output
Increased epinephrine secretion	Phaeochromocytoma
Decreased parasympathetic response	

means that a number of variables need to be considered, including those that influence filling and those that influence emptying.

Cardiac filling

Both ventricles are modulated by the same influences. The major factors that affect cardiac filling are the positive pressure in both the venous system and the ventricle. The former acts to push blood into the ventricle, aided at the end of diastole by a brief period of atrial systole, the only period of active ventricular filling. This is termed the ventricular filling pressure and is reflected in the right atrial pressure (RAP) for the right ventricle and the left atrial pressure (LAP) for the left ventricle. In the absence of tricuspid or mitral valve disease, the LAP equates to the end-diastolic pressure in the respective ventricular cavity. As we do not normally have a means of measuring direct LAP, in the absence of significant pulmonary disease, we take the pulmonary capillary wedge pressure (PCWP) as a surrogate for LAP and therefore LV end-diastolic pressure (see discussion on right heart catheterization in Chapter 6).

Filling pressures can be artificially increased by a fluid challenge, which can be demonstrated to increase CO for a short time. Filling pressures are also increased as a compensatory mechanism to preserve output in disease states. So RAP and PCWP may both be normal or increased in biventricular failure. Stressing the heart with exercise while undertaking a right heart catheter will usually demonstrate a rise in RAP or PCWP as the heart struggles to increase output. However, this is rarely performed as it is time consuming and cumbersome. In a pulmonary embolism or RV infarct, RAP may be high and PCWP may be low. In acute pulmonary oedema both may be high.

The RAP and PCWP reflect the preload of the heart (i.e. the volume of the ventricle at the end of diastole), and preload reducers such as nitrates vasodilate the venous system, increasing capacity and therefore reducing pressure. A consequence of this is lower forward flow into the ventricle. The relationship between increased ventricular filling (i.e. preload and CO) is known as Starling's law of the heart, beloved of medical students and examiners alike.

The positive pressure within the heart acts to impede the flow of blood into the heart, and gradually rises towards the end of diastole. When it exceeds the filling pressure generated in the right and left atria, the AV valves (mitral and tricuspid) will passively close. Conditions that increase the left and right ventricular diastolic pressure, such as stiff non-compliant ventricles, will impede blood entering the heart and reduce CO. A physiological marker of this is the right and left ventricular end-diastolic pressure (RVEDP and LVEDP). The LVEDP is routinely measured during a left ventriculogram and gives important information regarding the diastolic relaxation phase of the heart and therefore compliance of the ventricle.

Cardiac contraction

The passage of blood from the heart is dependent on a combination of force of contraction or contractility and the resistance to ventricular emptying (afterload).

- *Contractility*: This is governed, as ever, by a complex interdependency of various factors. But in a stable state, force of contraction is governed in the main by sympathetic drive, whether this is locally derived neuroendocrine norepinephrine or adrenally derived epinephrine. In the diseased heart, however, the ability to change the force of contraction is usually limited as the cardiac reserve is reduced. Some increase in force of contraction can be gained by increased stretch of the heart, although this is a short- to medium-term gain. This is an application of Starling's law, but only really becomes utilized when the force of contraction is limited in low output states (Table 2.2).
- *Peripheral vascular resistance/afterload*: When the heart contracts, it does so against a resistance that is derived from aortic valve opening (usually negligible in health) and the resistance arterioles of peripheral vascular beds. The degree of resistance of the arteriolar bed is very variable and under local paracrine, neuroendocrine and true endocrine control. A complex interplay of vasoconstrictors and

Table 2.2 Intrinsic and extrinsic factors that alter contractile state

Contractility increases with:	Beta-adrenergic receptors stimulated by norepinephrine released from nerve endings
	Circulating epinephrine
	Drugs such as ephedrine, digoxin and calcium
Contractility reduces with:	Acidosis
	Myocardial ischaemia
	Drugs such as beta-blockers, calcium channel blockers and antiarrhythmic agents

Table 2.3 Normal haemodynamic values

	Normal range (mmHg)	Definitely abnormal (mmHg)
Right atrium		
Mean	1–5	5+
a	2.5–7	7+
v	2–7.5	7.5+
Right ventricle		
Peak	17–32	32+
EDP	1–7	7+
Pulmonary artery		
Peak	17–32	32+
EDP	4–13	13+
PCWP	4.5–13	13+
Left atrium		
Mean	2–12	12+
a	4–16	16+
v	6–21	21+
Left ventricle		
Peak	90–140	140+
EDP	5–12	12+
Aorta		
Peak	90–140	140+
EDP	60–90	90+

a, arterial; v, venous; EDP, end-diastolic pressure; PCWP, pulmonary capillary wedge pressure.
Adapted from Kern MJ (ed.) *Cardiac Catheterization Handbook*. St Louis: Mosby, 1995.

vasodilators acts to change the resistance and hence flow through many different vascular beds. Occasionally single entities such as aortic stenosis, phaeochromocytomas secreting norepinephrine or renal artery stenosis can dramatically alter afterload.

Normal haemodynamic values are listed in Table 2.3.

Structural heart disease

This text is not the appropriate place to discuss in detail the anatomical complexities of congenital heart disease, especially cyanotic heart disease. However, it is appropriate to discuss those structural abnormalities that may present for the first time in adulthood:

- Patent foramen ovale
- Atrial septal defects
- Ventricular septal defects
- Patent ductus arteriosus.

Their angiographic assessment is discussed later.

Patent foramen ovale

An intermittently patent foramen ovale (PFO) may occur in up to 20 per cent of adults. In the newborn infant increased LAP, as blood passes through the lungs for the first time in any volume, effectively forces the septum primum against the septum secundum, closing the foramen ovale. The fusion of septum primum to secundum is usually complete by the first month after birth.

A PFO is not easily appreciated from the data acquired from the catheterization lab. The intermittent nature means that even a thorough right heart study with extensive saturation testing may still fail to pick it up and it is really a condition best diagnosed by echocardiography (either transthoracic or transoesophageal) with ancillary manoeuvres that raise RAP (cough or Valsalva). PFO shunting may be continuous left to right, or right to left with manoeuvres that increase RAP and the potential for right-to-left shunting may account for paradoxical embolus and stroke. This is a problem for patients who scuba dive, as they may well encounter increased right to left atrial pressure.

Atrial septal defects

ASDs fall into two main groups: the sinus venous defects and the secundum defects. These are difficult to see angiographically, but may be suggested by a full diagnostic saturation run during a right heart catheter (Figure 2.9).

Sinus venosus defects are formed by failure of fusion of the primitive inferior and superior vena cavae at their insertion into the right atrium, and if this involves an endocardial cushion defect, this is termed an ostium primum defect. They are more commonly located

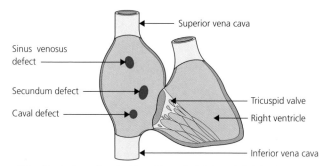

Figure 2.9   Typical anatomical location of atrial septal defects.

at the junction of RA and SVC, but can also occur at the junction of IVC and RA. They may also be accompanied by anomalous drainage of the right pulmonary veins, which normally drain into the left atrium next to the interatrial septum. If (partial) anomalous pulmonary venous drainage is present, then one of the right pulmonary veins may partially or completely drain into the RA, causing a step up in saturation.

A secundum ASD represents failure of closure of the foramen ovale, and is the most common form of ASD. They are visualized better by both transthoracic and transoesophageal echocardiography, and can be difficult to visualize on an angiographic study. Occasionally they may be seen on a late phase injection from a right-sided ventriculogram, which is then recorded as the bolus of contrast reforms in the LA, and may then flow back to the RA, but the image is rarely clear enough to make diagnosis possible by this method. More typically, anatomical definition is achieved by a venous catheter being used to cross the ASD and positioned in the right upper pulmonary vein. Injection here will opacify the LA and the shunt to RA. This is usually done in lateral or LAO cranial.

Ventricular septal defects

There are four major groups of ventricular septal defects (VSDs) that are seen presenting in adulthood, namely perimembranous, muscular, inlet and supracristal VSDs. AV defects usually present early and are not described here (Figure 2.10).

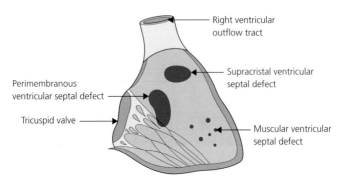

Figure 2.10   Typical anatomical location of ventricular septal defects.

PERIMEMBRANOUS VENTRICULAR SEPTAL DEFECTS

These are usually due to malalignment of the great vessels, and occur in the region immediately below the aortic valve. They usually discharge into the RV just below the tricuspid valve. They may be associated with aneurysm formation on the right side of the septum, which can lead to tricuspid valve dysfunction. Large defects can cause blood to be directed towards one or other of the great vessels.

MUSCULAR VENTRICULAR SEPTAL DEFECTS

These may be large and singular or multiple and small, but still cause haemodynamically significant shunting. This may be demonstrated at LV angiography as a 'cheesecloth type' picture, with many small defects being evident as contrast streams into the RV from the LV injection.

OUTLET OR SUPRACRISTAL VENTRICULAR SEPTAL DEFECTS

These are seen more often in Asian populations, and may be associated with AV regurgitation as well as the shunt. They discharge into the infundibulum just below the pulmonary valve. They are associated with an increased risk of progressive aortic valvular dysfunction.

PATENT DUCTUS ARTERIOSUS

The duct normally allows desaturated blood to pass from pulmonary artery to the placenta, via the aorta in the neonate. This closes rapidly and is converted to a fibrous ligament within the first few months of life. It originates from the anterior portion of the left pulmonary artery, within the first few centimetres of the LPA after the MPA bifurcation. It inserts into the inferior portion of the aortic arch, just beyond the origin of the right subclavian artery.

Anomalous and classical collateral vessels

Venous anomalies

PERSISTENT LEFT SUPERIOR VENA CAVA

This is a rare (<1 per cent) congenital malformation, that usually only becomes apparent when a placing a pacing lead from the left side is difficult. As an isolated defect it causes no shunting of blood left to right. There is failure of normal embryological development and instead of fusing with the right brachiocephalic vein, the left subclavian vein persists. It passes down the left lateral aspect of the heart, before inserting into the coronary sinus. The left brachiocephalic may remain as a small vestigial vessel, which can insert into the right brachiocephalic, and occasionally a pacing lead can be passed via that route. The increased flow of blood through the coronary sinus causes dilatation, which is obvious on TOE (Figure 2.11).

Anomalous arterial vessels

AORTIC ARCH ANOMALIES

Embryologically, six pairs of pharyngeal arch arteries develop sequentially and symmetrically with the corresponding branchial pouches. Some segments regress, but the third, fourth and sixth arches, along with the seventh intersegmental arteries and the left dorsal aorta persist, and form the normal aortic arch.

Normally, the left fourth arch becomes the aortic arch, the right fourth arch contributes to the brachiocephalic artery and the left dorsal aorta becomes the descending aorta. The dorsal intersegmental arteries bilaterally become the subclavian arteries.

A vascular ring is the term given to abnormal persistence of some segments and can be divided into three major types, but all may be

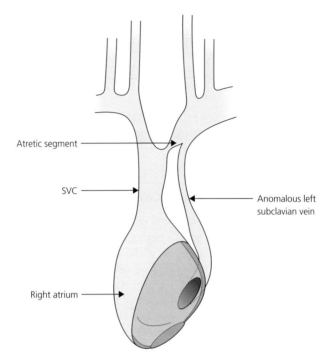

Figure 2.11 Anomalous left brachiocephalic vein.

complicated by atretic segments (segments completely blocked and present only as fibrous bands) (Figure 2.12):

- Double aortic arch
- Right arch with anomalous left subclavian artery
- Left arch with anomalous right subclavian artery.

The vascular ring may encircle the trachea or oesophagus, causing partial obstruction of either/both, as the aberrant subclavian, left or right usually runs behind the oesophagus. The partially reabsorbed atretic segments remain, completing the sling. They can be seen at aortography, but need to be delineated by CT/CMR.

The left arch with anomalous right subclavian can cause problems for the radial operator.

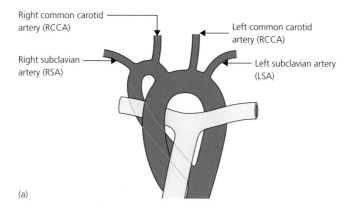

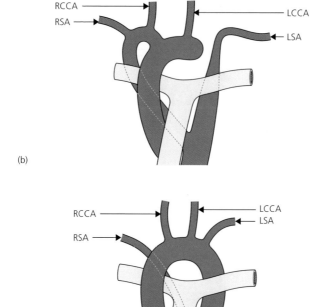

Figure 2.12 Aortic arch anomalies. (a) Double aortic arch. (b) Right-sided aortic arch with anomalous left subclavian artery. (c) Left-sided aortic arch with anomalous right subclavian artery.

Coronary arteries

LEFT MAIN STEM

There are four major abnormalities of the LMS [1]. They occur when the LMS arises from the right coronary sinus, and are termed the anterior, septal, intra-arterial and retroaortic courses (Figure 2.13). The right and left coronary arteries may have a single origin, but this is not always the case. The LMS may also arise from the posterior sinus, but

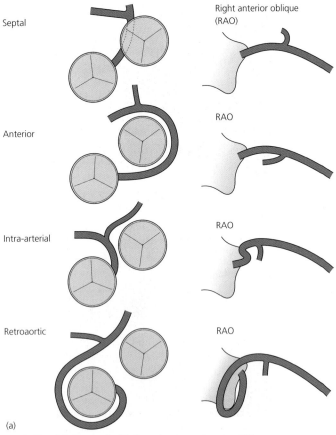

(a)

Figure 2.13 (a) Congenital left main stem abnormalities.

this is apparent from the RAO caudal view, with a posteriorly directed catheter.

- *Septal course*: The LMS arises from the right coronary sinus and courses initially in the muscular septum, where it gives off a Cx branch in the mid-septum. This then has to take a sweeping curve

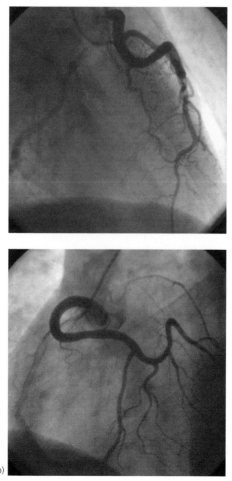

(b)

Figure 2.13   (b) Angiographic images of aberrant left main stem from right coronary sinus (anterior route).

backward to take on a more traditional path in the AV groove. In an RAO 30° view, this is seen as quite a straight take off, with a Cx that appears above the line of the LAD, making a curve retrogradely. This is usually benign.

- *Anterior course*: This variation crosses the anterior free wall of the RV in front of the pulmonary artery. It follows a predominantly epicardial course, before giving both Cx and LAD in a more distal position. The Cx again takes a retrograde course to achieve a position in the AV groove, but in this case appears to pass below the line of the LM/LAD in the RAO 30° view. It is benign.
- *Interarterial course*: This is not a benign anomaly, as the LMS is subject to external compression and there is a risk of sudden death. The LMS arises from the right sinus and immediately takes a leftward direction, passing between the aorta and pulmonary trunks. It then arrives at a more traditional location and the LAD and Cx follow their normal course. On the RAO 30° angiogram the interarterial segment is seen as a short upward turn, with normal LAD and Cx position (i.e. no retrograde section of Cx seen).
- *Retroaortic course*: The LMS passes posteriorly in a loop around the aortic root, it then gives off Cx in a near normal position. It is seen as the only LMS anomaly that passes inferoposteriorly. It is essentially benign.

LEFT ANTERIOR DESCENDING

The LAD may arise from the right coronary sinus or the RCA directly. It is described as following the same courses as the LMS: septal, anterior, interarterial and retroaortic. Angiographically they look the same, but the clues gained from the Cx location, differentiating the septal and anterior courses are absent. The only dangerous aberrant LAD is the one following an interarterial course.

CIRCUMFLEX

The most common anomaly is the Cx arising from the right coronary sinus. It may arise either from the RCA as a very proximal branch, or as a separate origin, and is benign. Rarely it may arise from the posterior sinus.

A Cx anomaly can be missed angiographically if the LCA has a large early diagonal, which may be mistaken for the Cx. If the Cx territory is only sparsely supplied and the RCA not very dominant, then an aberrant Cx is likely. If it arises as a separate branch it may be difficult to engage. If the aberrant Cx is a very early branch, then engaging the vessel may actually put the catheter tip past the origin of the Cx which may then not be appreciated.

A retroaortic course is appreciated by the posterior course of the vessel and the end-on vessel seen as a dot posteriorly to the aortic root on the left ventriculogram.

RIGHT CORONARY ARTERY

The most common RCA abnormality is the anteriorly arising RCA, originating from the right sinus. Catheter selection is difficult to advise upon, but typically a JR4, Williams or AL1 will facilitate cannulation in most cases. It is possible to engage an aberrant RCA arising in the left coronary sinus with Judkins 5 or 6 or Amplatz 2 or 3 catheters.

An anomalous RCA can also arise from the posterior or left coronary sinuses. It has been reported to arise as an early branch of the left main. It will typically take an interarterial course between pulmonary artery and the aorta to gain its normal position. This course places it at risk of compression and is not benign.

Collaterals

- *Kugel's artery*: This collateral vessel connects the sinoatrial artery to the AV nodal artery, and provides critical collateral support to the PD artery in the presence of an RCA or Cx occlusion, depending on vessel dominance (Figure 2.14). It runs through the atrial septum.
- *Circle of Vieussens*: This is a collateral that runs between the conus branch of the RCA and a proximal RV branch of the LAD. It is of value in proximal LAD occlusion.
- *Coronary arcade*: This collateral is occasionally patent even in the absence of occlusive coronary disease. It connects distal Cx with distal RCA, and flow can be in either direction depending on which epicardial artery occludes. Another arcade exists between distal LAD and PD arteries. Figure 2.15 shows an occluded RCA receiving collaterals from AV groove vessel arising from a non-dominant Cx. Figure 2.16 shows an apical arcade from a dominant RCA to an occluded LAD.

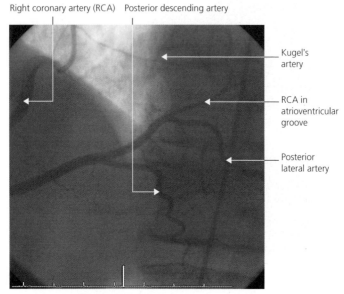

Right coronary artery (RCA)   Posterior descending artery

Kugel's artery

RCA in atrioventricular groove

Posterior lateral artery

Figure 2.14 Kugel's artery.

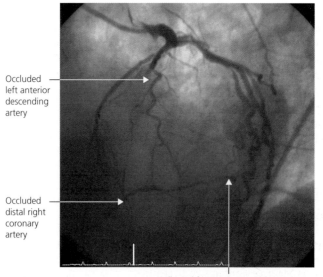

Occluded left anterior descending artery

Occluded distal right coronary artery

Collateral from atrioventricular groove circumflex to right coronary artery

Figure 2.15 Collaterals from circumflex to right coronary artery.

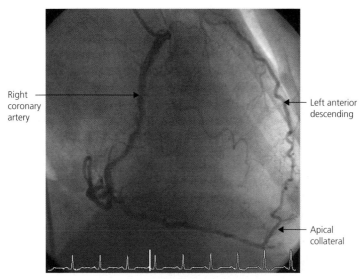

Figure 2.16 Collaterals from posterior descending artery to left anterior decending artery.

- *Septals*: This important source of collaterals can protect either the LAD or RCA, depending on which vessel has the disease. For example the gradually progressive limitation of antegrade flow through a LAD may encourage septal arteries to open up, collateralizing the LAD via the PD artery. Obviously the collateral flow can run in the opposite direction. This is shown in Figure 2.17 where the septal collaterals can be clearly seen, although the LAD is ghosting, a phase which suggests that contrast is just seen in the vessel.

Cardiac surgical procedures in grown up congenital heart (GUCH) patients

Fontan procedure

François Maurice Fontan was a twentieth-century French cardiac surgeon who described an operation to divert systemic venous blood directly to the pulmonary artery, effectively bypassing the RV. This has

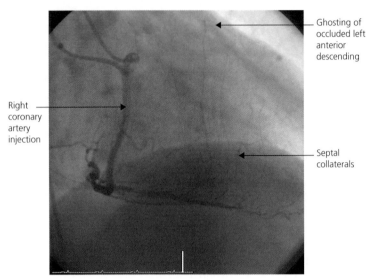

Figure 2.17   Collaterals via septal arteries.

a role in tricuspid atresia, hypoplastic right heart and single ventricle. Initially this was achieved by sewing the RA appendage to the RPA, but evolved into either direct SVC to superior RPA or a conduit from IVC to RPA or MPA. The conduit may run either inside or outside the RA. The major complication is pulmonary hypertension or focal pulmonary artery stenosis, both of which are poor prognostic signs.

Classic and bidirectional Glenn

William Glenn was a twentieth-century American cardiac surgeon, who described a direct connection between the SVC and the RPA, which was disconnected from the MPA, allowing upper body venous blood to run directly into the right lung, bypassing the RA/RV. This evolved into the bidirectional Glenn, which did not disarticulate the RPA from the MPA. Its original role was as a palliative procedure for tricuspid atresia. Angiographically, the state of the shunt is examined from a direct SVC injection, although it is probably much better assessed by CMR.

Blalock–Taussig shunt

This is the surgical connection of the subclavian artery to the pulmonary artery, which augments pulmonary flow in restrictive congenital heart disease. The conduit is either mobilized subclavian or a synthetic graft. It is a palliative procedure. The residual quality of the shunt can be assessed by arch aortography or selective subclavian injection.

Mustard procedure

This operation was used to treat transposition of the great arteries by directing vena caval inflow into the LV. This is because the anatomical LV is connected to the pulmonary outflow tract and is carrying deoxygenated blood to the lungs. Similarly, pulmonary venous blood is directed into the RV because the RV is connected to the aorta and therefore pumping oxygenated blood. It consisted of a pericardial baffle which incorporated the insertion of both caval insertions (inferior and superior) and the mitral valve, thus directing deoxygenated blood into the LV. The pulmonary vein insertions were excluded from the baffle and therefore oxygenated blood could only enter the RV cavity and therefore move into the systemic circulation.

The Mustard procedure is complicated by RV dysfunction, progressive tricuspid regurgitation, SVC obstruction and atrial arrythmias. Isolated pulmonary vein obstruction can also occur, causing segmental pulmonary oedema. Angiography is useful only for demonstrating leaks from the baffle, which cause left to right shunting. Cross-sectional imaging is probably the way forward.

Arterial switch

This operation consists of transection of the aorta and pulmonary arteries above the sinus region, and anastamosis of the ascending aorta to the pulmonary sinus and vice versa. The coronary arteries are resected and reimplanted to the pulmonary artery.

Ross procedure

This describes the removal of the native pulmonary valve and placing it in the aortic area. A homograft is then placed in the pulmonary area, where the pressure and therefore wear and tear is likely to be less. Echo follow-up is more appropriate.

Further reading

Baim Donald S and Grossman William (eds). *Grossman's Cardiac Catheterization, Angiography, and Intervention*, 6th edn. Philadelphia: Lippincott Williams & Wilkins, 2000.

Gosling JA, Harris PF, Humpherson JR, Whitmore I. Willan PLT. *Atlas of Human Anatomy*. Edinburgh: Churchill Livingstone, 1985.

Kern MJ (ed.) *Cardiac Catheterization Handbook*, 2nd edn. St Louis: Mosby, 1995.

Yale University School of Medicine. *Congenital Heart Disease* www. med.yale.edu/intmed/cardio/chd/contents/index.html.

Reference

1. Serota H, Barth CW, III, Seuc CA *et al.* Rapid identification of the course of anomalous coronary arteries in adults: the 'dot and eye' method. *Am J Cardiol* 1990; **65**: 891–898.

Transradial access 3

Historical perspectives

Catheterization of the heart via upper limb access sites has a long history, and has played a pivotal role in the development of invasive cardiology. The first catheterization of a human heart was performed in 1929 when Werner Forssmann cut down on his own left antecubital vein and inserted a ureteric catheter which he then advanced to his right atrium. In the late 1950s Mason Sones performed the first selective coronary angiograms using a surgical technique to expose and cannulate the brachial artery, and the era of modern invasive and interventional cardiology began.

These upper limb access techniques require considerable surgical expertise to identify, dissect out, cannulate and repair the selected vessels, and this limited the widespread application of cardiac catheterization. In 1962, however, HJ Ricketts and HL Abrams employed a percutaneous transfemoral approach to simplify the arterial access component of cardiac catheterization procedures. In 1967 Melvin Judkins developed a series of preshaped catheters to further simplify transfemoral procedures. With these two developments upper limb access sites were largely abandoned, and the majority of cardiologists performed procedures via the femoral artery. Undoubtedly, these advances in femoral access techniques facilitated an explosive growth in procedures that would not have been possible if cardiologists had remained reliant on technically demanding surgical approaches to upper limb access sites. It seemed clear at this time that brachial access would be reserved for a very small number of patients with contraindications to the use of the femoral artery.

Femoral and brachial access site complications

Performing cardiac procedures via the femoral or brachial arteries does have important disadvantages. Both vessels are end arteries that are situated close to major nerves and veins. Because of this unfavourable neurovascular anatomy, access site complications can have major life- or limb-threatening consequences. The risk of major femoral or brachial access site complications is substantially increased when intensive antithrombotic regimes are employed (Figure 3.1). Contemporary data indicate that important femoral access complications occur in around 1 per cent of simple procedures, with a sharp rise to almost 20 per cent when complex procedures are performed in the setting of intensive antithrombotic therapy [1–4].

These femoral access site problems have not been solved by vascular access closure devices. Although they can decrease the time required

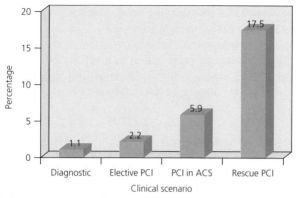

Figure 3.1 Femoral access site complications in contemporary practice. PCI, percutaneous intervention; MI, myocardial infarction; ACS, acute coronary syndrome.

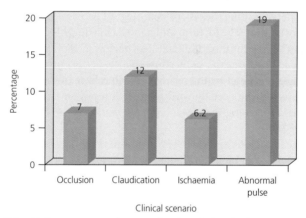

Figure 3.2 Major neurovascular complications in brachial cutdown procedures.

to achieve haemostasis, a recent meta-analysis of 4000 patients in randomized trials demonstrated an increased rate of femoral access site complications when these devices are employed [5]. Skilled high-volume operators can achieve low complication rates when a surgical approach to the brachial artery is employed, even in the setting of intensive antithrombotic therapy. For less skilled or infrequent operators, most series consistently report a 5–10 per cent incidence of major complications [6–9] (Figure 3.2). These brachial access problems have not been consistently solved by the use of a technically simpler percu-taneous approach to the brachial artery [10].

Because of these high complication rates, a surgical or percutaneous brachial approach is not a viable option for most cardiologists. This high rate of debilitating femoral and brachial complications prompted cardi-ologists to search for alternative safer access sites.

Principles of transradial access

The radial artery has been safely employed for many years for haemo-dynamic monitoring. It is an attractive access site for cardiac proce-dures because of its favourable neurovascular anatomy. The radial artery has a superficial course at the wrist, which facilitates percuta-neous puncture. The artery overlies the forearm bones, facilitating compression haemostasis. No major nerves or veins lie close to the radial artery, limiting the risk of neurological damage or arteriovenous fistula formation. The forearm and hand have a dual blood supply, with the ulnar artery limiting the risk of ischaemic complications if radial artery occlusion occurs as a consequence of the procedure. These advantages are offset by the relatively small calibre of the radial artery, which precluded its use for cardiac procedures when only large calibre catheterization equipment was available between the late 1950s and mid-1980s.

In the late 1980s and early 1990s, advances in materials science and engineering technology facilitated the production of catheterization equipment that was compatible with introduction into the relatively small-calibre radial artery. These developments coincided with an explosive rise in the rate of femoral complications associated with the introduction of coronary stents. These two factors led cardiologists to evaluate the use of the radial artery as an access site for diagnostic and therapeutic cardiac procedures. Campeau reported the first series of diag-nostic cardiac catheterizations performed via the radial artery in 1989 [11] with Kiemeneij and colleagues reporting the first interventional series in 1995 [12,13]. The first large-scale transradial interventional programme in the UK was established at the University Hospital of North Staffordshire in Stoke in 1998 [14]. A series of randomized trials have compared radial and femoral access, with a recent meta-analysis confirming that the radial approach reduces access site complications and is therefore safer [15]. The prevention of access site complications reduces costs by 10–15 per cent [16]. The easy application of a local compression device to the radial puncture site facilitates immediate ambulation and improves quality of life [16]. In direct comparative studies, the majority of patients who have an option will prefer radial over femoral access [16].

Transradial access does have some disadvantages. The radial artery is a small-calibre vessel which is prone to spasm, and variations in the anatomy of the arm or head and neck vessels can pose unexpected challenges. Because of these technical challenges there is an important learning curve associated with the use of radial access. Technical advances in the production of the equipment specifically designed for transradial use, along with increasing operator experience has simplified and optimized the technique, and all competent femoral operators can become safe effective radial operators if they devote the time required to overcome the learning curve.

Anatomical issues

Normal anatomy

Transradial operators need to be familiar with the vascular anatomy of the upper limb vessels. Figures 3.3 and 3.4 illustrate the relevant arterial anatomy of a normal individual. The first branch of the ascending aorta is the brachiocephalic artery, which divides into the right common carotid and subclavian arteries. The subclavian artery passes under the clavicle to become the axillary artery, which becomes the brachial artery as it enters the upper arm. Close to the elbow joint the brachial artery divides into the radial and ulnar arteries. The radial artery passes on the lateral margin of the forearm towards the wrist, with the ulnar artery passing down the medial margin of the forearm. The ulnar artery is often a large vessel, but since it is deeper lying, more mobile and lies close to the ulnar nerve it is not as suitable for use as a common access site. In the upper forearm the radial artery lies below muscle bodies, and is not palpable. In the lower forearm the artery emerges from below the forearm muscles and lies superficially over the distal end of the radius bone. At the lower end of the forearm, just distal to the styloid process palpable on the lateral border of the lower forearm, the radial and ulnar arteries divide into two branches that enter the hand and anastomose to form the superficial and deep palmar arches.

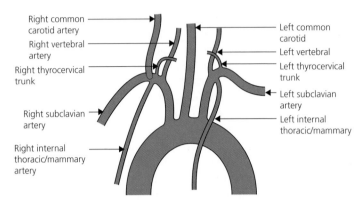

Figure 3.3 Vascular anatomy of the aortic arch and proximal head and neck vessels.

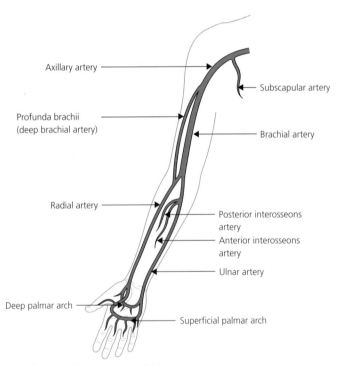

Figure 3.4 Vascular anatomy of the arm.

In most individuals the radial artery at the wrist is 2.5–3.0 mm in diameter, and is easily compatible with 6F or larger sheath sizes. In around 10 per cent of individuals (particularly elderly females, individuals of short stature or diabetics) the artery is less than 2.5 mm in diameter, and use of smaller systems may be required if discomfort or difficulty is encountered with attempted insertion of a larger calibre sheath.

Anatomical variation

In around 10% of patients variation in the anatomy of the upper limb arterial system occurs. In the majority of these patients the anatomical variations are relatively minor, cause no difficulty to the operator and are therefore undetected. In a proportion of cases a more extreme anatomical variation occurs leading to procedural difficulty. Although these peripheral anatomical difficulties can often be overcome by a skilled operator, they are a major cause of access failure. The most frequent important anomaly is tortuosity or a 360° loop in the radial [17]. These tortuous segments and loops can be traversed with a suitable wire (a hydrophilic angioplasty wire is usually suitable), which straightens the affected segment and allows subsequent catheter passage. These manoeuvres, however, can initiate marked radial spasm which may prevent catheter passage. In this situation we recommend selecting an alternative access site to avoid further discomfort.

In around 1/100 individuals the radial artery arises in the upper arm from the axillary or brachial artery. If the aberrant radial vessel is large, there will be no problems during the procedure. If the aberrant vessel is small, spasm is easily provoked, and the occurrence of discomfort in the upper arm provoked by catheter exchange is a clue that the operator is working in one of these small aberrant arteries. This problem can usually be overcome by administering vasodilators and/or changing to a smaller calibre catheter. When these aberrant vessels are very small they allow the passage of a guidewire but can be easily ruptured if a catheter is forcefully advanced. There are a large number of other rare variations in the anatomy of the forearm vessels. If angiography demonstrates that a complex anatomical variation is present, conversion to another access site may be required.

In the elderly or in association with hypertension the subclavian or brachiocephalic artery may become tortuous. In these patients use of a hydrophilic wire in association with deep inspiration may allow entry to the aorta; an exchange length guidewire should then be used when changing catheters to minimize the risk of subsequently re-crossing these areas. In patients with widespread vascular disease, unexpected atheromatous stenoses or occlusions in the subclavian or brachiocephalic vessels (which are frequently bilateral) occur. In elderly or hypertensive individuals the aortic arch is frequently unfolded (Figure 3.5). This directs the origin of the brachiocephalic artery into a more posterior position, and wire or catheter entry into the ascending aorta is compromised. A deep inspiration will often realign the brachiocephalic and ascending aorta, allowing catheter entry or manipulation.

Variations in the anatomy of the head and neck vessel origins from the aorta are rare. The commonest of these variations is a retro-oesophageal subclavian origin (incidence 1/400), which is a partial vascular ring or aortic arch anomaly [18]. In this situation the right subclavian artery passes behind the oesophagus and joins the upper descending aorta. In these patients catheter manipulation is difficult, and only experienced operators will be able to successfully complete the procedure.

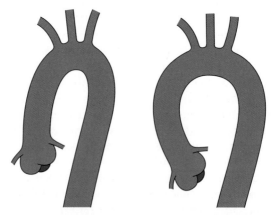

Figure 3.5   Normal (left) and unfolded (right) aortic arch. In patients with an unfolded arch catheter passage from brachiocephalic into ascending aorta requires that catheter is manipulated anteriorly from the brachiocephalic before the ascending aorta can be entered, increasing technical complexity.

Patient assessment, laboratory set-up and radial artery cannulation

Patient selection

We recommend using the right radial approach in most patients, since catheterization laboratories are usually optimally configured for operators standing at the patient's right hand side. For an experienced operator, there are few absolute contraindications. Many operators use a bedside test of the hand's collateral circulation before proceeding with a transradial procedure. This can be a simple modified Allen test, or a more objective test using an oximeter [19,20].

To perform an Allen test the radial and ulnar arteries are simultaneously occluded by manual compression (Figure 3.6), whilst the patient flexes and extends their fingers, leading to the induction of ischaemia in the hand, which appears pale and blanched. Whilst maintaining radial compression, ulnar compression is then released. In around 95 per cent of individuals, the palm will flush with blood within 10 seconds (with an unfavourable result being more common in the elderly) [14,21]. This favourable Allen test result suggests that adequate non-radial based perfusion of the hand is available in the event of an iatrogenic radial artery occlusion, and it is therefore safe to perform a transradial procedure.

An initially unfavourable Allen test is not proof that the hand is dependent on a single arterial source. The relative flow in radial and ulnar arteries can be varied autonomically, and the anatomical basis for establishment of an adequate collateral circulation will be present in most patients with an initially unfavourable clinical test [22]. In patients with an unfavourable clinical Allen test, further evaluation with pulse oximetry is indicated [20]. A pulse oximeter is positioned on the thumb, demonstrating phasic flow of highly saturated arterial blood. The radial artery is then occluded by manual compression for 2 minutes. If a normal phasic flow of saturated blood persists, a patent palmar arch is present. If pulsatile flow is initially abolished, but returns within 2 minutes, an adequate recruitable collateral circulation is present. In both of these situations, radial catheterization is safe. If pulsatile flow is abolished by radial compression and does not reappear, there is a risk of ischaemia if radial occlusion occurs.

A bilaterally unfavourable oximeter test is present in only 1.5 per cent of individuals (most commonly older males). Because of the risk of thumb ischaemia in the event of an iatrogenic radial artery occlusion,

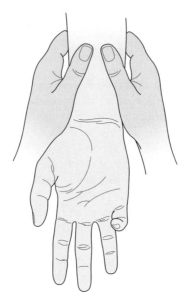

Figure 3.6 Application of simultaneous radial and ulnar compression to perform an Allen test.

an alternative access site should be employed for these patients. The only other relative contraindication to a radial approach would be the presence of end-stage chronic renal failure. These patients may require the construction of a forearm arteriovenous fistula to facilitate haemodialysis, and it is important that their upper limb vessels are not cannulated.

Patient and catheter laboratory preparation

A full explanation of the radial procedure should be provided before the patient enters the catheterization laboratory, stressing the safety of the access site and the capacity to mobilize immediately. Patients should be warned that they will experience some discomfort in the wrist with local anaesthetic administration, and that vasodilator cocktails (if used) will induce a hot feeling in the hand and arm. During the learning curve it is wise to insert an intravenous cannula in the opposite arm. An intravenous saline infusion should be prepared, and 1.2 mg of atropine drawn up before commencing the procedure so that vasovagal reactions can be easily and rapidly dealt with.

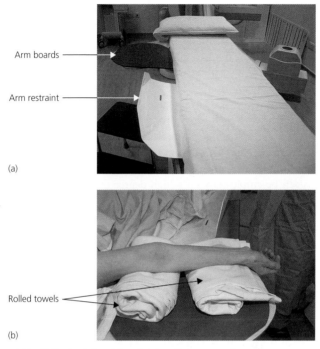

Arm boards

Arm restraint

(a)

Rolled towels

(b)

Figure 3.7 Catheter lab set for right radial approach.

The precise table set-up varies between operators and institutions. At the University Hospital of North Staffordshire we use two overlapping arm boards to allow the abducted arm to be supported and extended at the wrist and elbow on two rolled-up towels. An arm restraint is positioned further along the table to provide the operators with a suitable flat working area (Figure 3.7). The wrist is cleaned and the patient draped with sterile towels. If there is no contraindication, two puffs of sublingual glyceryl trinitrate (GTN) are administered to increase radial artery calibre and aid cannulation.

Radial artery puncture technique

A wide range of dedicated transradial cannulation equipment is available. Some specific radial puncture systems (produced by Kimmal and Terumo) consist of a soft short cannula mounted on a small-calibre needle that communicates with an observation chamber. When the needle punctures the radial artery, blood flashes back into the observation chamber and the cannula is then inserted into the radial artery. The cannula is then used to administer a vasodilator cocktail, and a guidewire is introduced into the artery. The cannula is then withdrawn and the radial sheath inserted over the guidewire.

These systems have two advantages. The vasodilator cocktail is administered prior to wire or sheath entry into the radial artery, which may reduce the risk of inducing spasm. If there is any difficulty in advancing the guidewire, the short introducer cannula allows arm angiography to be easily performed, facilitating problem solving. These radial cannulation systems can be employed with a high degree of success, but do have a learning curve of their own. Femoral trained operators are very familiar with an open needle Seldinger-based technique for arterial cannulation. Because of this, using a modified open needle technique for radial cannulation is usually easier to master. It is advisable to use a specific radial puncture kit to access the artery. Radial puncture needles are short and small calibre, and often have a flat-sided hub. These features help the operator to easily manipulate the needle. These radial needles are supplied with a guidewire optimized for radial cannulation. The tip of the wire is usually soft to facilitate atraumatic entry into the radial artery. The shaft of the wire is considerably stiffer to aid in tracking the sheath into the artery.

When the patient is prepared and draped, the radial artery is identified by palpation. Some operators prefer to puncture the artery with the table at a low height and the operator comfortably positioned on a stool. Other operators prefer to stand with the table elevated to its maximum height, avoiding the need to bend over the puncture site. The table height setting and use of a stool should be experimented with to identify a personal preference. The artery is usually palpable over several centimetres, from the base of the thumb to the mid forearm. In this situation a well pulsating site 1–2 cm proximal to the styloid process is usually the optimal position to puncture the radial artery. More distal punctures around the wrist skin creases are often difficult as the artery is smaller, more tortuous, and lies partially below the fibrous flexor retinaculum. More proximal punctures can be difficult as the artery lies in a deeper position. If the artery is only palpable in a small area, a distal or proximal puncture may be unavoidable.

A small volume of local anaesthetic (1–2 mL of 2 per cent lignocaine (lidocaine)) is infiltrated into the skin over the planned puncture site.

Deep infiltration or use of a larger volume of local anaesthetic should be avoided, as this may induce spasm or prevent palpation of the pulse. The puncture site and proximal artery are palpated by the non-dominant hand, and the needle is introduced at a 30° angle to the skin (Figure 3.8). The skin entry point selected should be directly above the planned arterial puncture site. The radial artery usually lies only a millimetre or two below the skin surface, and arterial blood will flow back from the needle hub when the anterior wall of the artery is punctured. Because the puncture needle is small calibre, the operator will not see the vigorous pulsatile flow that accompanies puncture of a femoral artery with a large-calibre needle. A low-volume, less pulsatile bleed back is evidence of satisfactory puncture.

The needle position is then fixed with the non-dominant hand, and the guidewire is introduced. If the wire will not easily exit from the tip of the needle, it is important not to attempt to forcefully advance it against resistance. The wire should be removed and the needle position

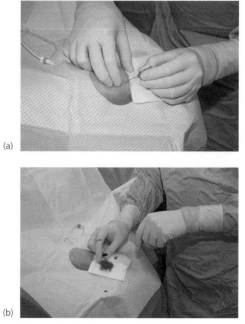

(a)

(b)

Figure 3.8 Radial cannulation by open needle. (a) Puncture with Seldinger open needle; (b) insertion of guidewire.

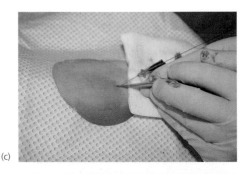

(c)

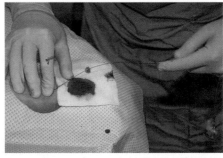

(d)

Figure 3.8 (c) skin incision; (d) remove needle and insert sheath. This figure shows a left-handed operator. Right-handed operators should palpate the artery with the left hand and puncture with the right hand.

adjusted before further attempts at wire introduction. Usually, this difficulty occurs because the needle bevel is partially embedded in the posterior wall of the artery, and slightly withdrawing the needle will facilitate easy guidewire entry. If the wire enters the artery with no difficulty but resistance is encountered in the mid or upper forearm, the wire has usually entered a small side branch. Withdrawal (for 1–2 cm) and rotation of the wire will usually allow satisfactory wire advancement.

A scalpel is then used to make a small incision in the skin at the wire entry point. This is to facilitate sheath introduction, and is particularly important when 6F or larger sheaths are required. Following this the sheath is usually easily inserted over the wire.

Specific radial access sheaths are available, and should be used in all cases. The dilators on radial systems are very tapered and the sheaths usually have a hydrophilic coating. These two features facilitate sheath introduction into the small-calibre muscular radial artery. During the learning curve long (23 cm) sheaths are often employed. These long sheaths minimize the risk of inducing spasm related to excessive catheter torquing manoeuvres, but have the disadvantage of sometimes being difficult to remove. For experienced radial operators short (7 or 11 cm) sheaths are usually satisfactory as catheter manipulation is reduced and spasm less likely. These short sheaths are less traumatic for the radial artery. When a short sheath is used, it is important to secure the sheath to the skin (usually with transparent cannula dressings) to prevent accidental sheath withdrawal during catheter exchanges.

Radial artery spasm is more likely when large-calibre sheaths are used (as is postprocedural radial occlusion) [23,24]. For this reason we recommend using 5F sheath systems for diagnostic angiography and selected simple angioplasty procedures, with larger calibre systems reserved predominantly for more complex interventional procedures.

Most operators administer some form of vasodilator/antithrombotic cocktail at this stage. There is some published data available to guide the optimal make-up of these cocktails. The data available relating to heparin administration suggest that the rate of procedure-related radial artery occlusion is reduced if heparin is administered [25], and other studies indicate that a combination of nitrates and calcium antagonists reduce the risk of radial spasm [26]. On this basis some operators administer a cocktail of heparin (2500 u for diagnostic procedures, 5000 u for PCI), nitrate (200 μg GTN) and calcium antagonist (2.5 mg of verapamil) made up to 10 mL with saline and given as a rapid injection into the sheath. This type of cocktail is most useful in the learning curve when the risk of spasm is highest. Its disadvantage is the risk of systematic effects (bradycardia and hypotension) and the induction of an unpleasant hot sensation in the hand and arm related to rapid vasodilatation and the low pH of the heparin. Aspirating 2 or 3 mL of blood into the cocktail syringe allows the ph of the solution to equalise to that of blood, reducing the ph mediated component of the burning sensation.

Experienced operators often dispense with the vasodilators and give the heparin centrally via a catheter positioned in the aorta, minimizing the risk of systemic hypotension or bradycardia and avoiding the hot flush in the hand. After secure sheath insertion the patient's arm is adducted to a position alongside the body. This adducted position, in combination with the use of an arm restraint, allows the operators to rest equipment on a flat area of the table.

Catheterization technique

Catheter selection

For diagnostic purposes, 5F catheters provide a good balance between catheter performance and ease of use. The catheter lumen is of sufficient size to allow easy contrast injection, the torque response and kink resistance is satisfactory, and the small external catheter diameter limits radial distension (thereby limiting the risk of spasm induction) and allows a 5F sheath to be used. Before catheter insertion the patient's left hand is placed behind their head, to facilitate image acquisition (if the arm is moved after catheter insertion, it may dislodge the catheter). Catheters must always be introduced and removed over a guidewire, avoiding forceful wire or catheter advancement. This will minimize the risk of trauma to the brachial, axillary or brachiocephalic arteries. Catheters are advanced up the arm under fluoroscopic control to ensure that the wire tracks in the correct direction. If any difficulty is experienced in advancing or exchanging catheters or wires, an angiogram should be obtained via the sheath to delineate the cause of the difficulty. If the wire does not enter the aorta easily, a deep inspiration by the patient will straighten the orientation of the brachiocephalic vessel and usually allow entry. If significant tortuosity is present in the arm or head and neck vessels, a hydrophilic guidewire will usually track more easily than a conventional guidewire.

For diagnostic angiography there are a number of approaches to catheter selection. Many operators have used Judkins left and right catheters and a pigtail with a high success rate. The disadvantage to this approach is that the catheters were not designed to be used from the right arm, and their performance is therefore compromised, particularly that of the Judkins left catheter. Other operators have reported good success rates using Amplatz left catheters to image both coronary arteries, thereby reducing the number of catheters required [16]. For inexperienced operators there is an increased risk of coronary dissection (particularly in the right coronary artery) associated with this catheter, and this has limited its uptake. Traditional multipurpose catheters were often used by brachial operators, and allow coronary and left ventricular angiography to be performed with a single catheter. Many femoral operators have little experience with these catheters, and they are therefore not widely used.

We recommend using a diagnostic angiographic catheter designed specifically for the right radial approach. The Terumo Tiger catheter

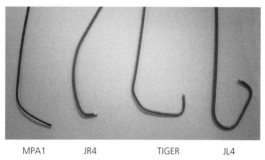

MPA1   JR4   TIGER   JL4

Figure 3.9 Preferred cardiac catheters for radial procedures.

has a configuration similar to an unfolded Judkins left catheter (Figure 3.9). The catheter is advanced to the mid ascending aorta over a guidewire, stopping well above the left coronary ostium. The wire is removed, the catheter is flushed and pressure monitoring established. The image intensifier is placed in the left anterior oblique (LAO) position to optimize visualization during catheter manipulation. The catheter is then advanced down the aorta with clockwise rotation. In the majority of individuals this manoeuvre will gently engage the left main coronary artery. After acquisition of the left coronary images the intensifier is returned to the LAO projection and the catheter is gently withdrawn from the left main coronary artery. In many patients the Tiger catheter can now be advanced and rotated into the right coronary sinus, allowing engagement of the right coronary artery and obviating the need for a catheter exchange.

It is important to note that this manoeuvre can be difficult to accomplish, and that the catheter tip has a tendency to point superiorly and selectively engage the conus branch. If optimal right coronary engagement is not easily and rapidly achieved we recommend changing to a Judkins right four catheter, which engages the right coronary artery in a fashion familiar to femoral operators using clockwise rotation in the LAO projection.

Graft angiography

For patients with a history of cardiac surgery, venous grafts can be easily cannulated from the right arm, but the left internal mammary artery (LIMA) presents a problem. Some authors have reported subselective angiography of the LIMA from the right arm by cannulating the left subclavian and injecting contrast with a blood pressure cuff inflated in the left arm. Images obtained with this type of technique are often sub-optimal and we do not advocate this approach. These patients can be investigated using a left radial approach in most cases. The LIMA is usually easily intubated with a Judkins right four or LIMA catheter. Obtaining images of the LIMA from the left arm is usually technically simple. Femoral operators often have to overcome considerable technical challenges to enter the left subclavian in patients with atheromatous aortas, and these issues are circumvented by the use of a left radial approach. For venous grafts, a Judkins right four, left or right coronary bypass catheter or an Amplatz left catheter can be used in conventional fashion. Catheter manipulation and angiographic projections are identical to those employed for a femoral approach.

Ventriculography

For ventriculography, we recommend using a pigtail catheter. Crossing the aortic valve with a pigtail catheter inserted from the right arm can sometimes be surprisingly difficult. When a pigtail catheter is advanced into the ascending aorta from the right arm, it frequently enters the right coronary sinus, with the tip below the valve orifice. In order to cross the valve, the guidewire should be withdrawn and a loop formed with the tip. As the catheter is then slowly further withdrawn, the wire is advanced down the catheter, usually causing the tip to prolapse through the valve. After acquisition of the ventriculogram, it is important to pay attention to two aspects of the pigtail catheter withdrawal. When pulling back the catheter to record the transaortic gradient, the catheter should be withdrawn for the minimum distance required to obtain the pressure measurements. If the catheter is rapidly withdrawn for a long distance, the looped tip of the pigtail catheter will enter the brachiocephalic or subclavian vessels with a potential risk of vascular injury. When pressure monitoring is complete, the guidewire must be reinserted into the pigtail catheter prior to removal, or the looped end of the catheter may traumatize the head and neck or arm vessels during withdrawal.

The left radial approach

Some operators preferentially use the left radial approach. The radial cannulation technique is identical to the description for right radial access. From the left arm catheters enter the aortic arch in a relatively distal position. The orientation and behaviour of catheters in the ascending aorta is therefore very similar to catheters introduced from the femoral artery. The technique for selecting and manipulating catheters introduced from the left radial is identical to and therefore very familiar to femoral operators, reducing learning curve issues. The reason that most operators prefer a right radial approach relates to the configuration of catheterization laboratories, which are designed around the principle of operators standing on the patient's right hand side. This requires that left radial operators stand on the left side after puncture, often in a confined space with the monitors usually in a sub-optimal position. As an alternative the arm can be adducted across the abdomen after puncture, to allow the operators to work on the patient's right, which can be uncomfortable for the patient or operators (Figure 3.10). For the majority of operators these disadvantages outweigh the simplified catheter manipulation, and the right radial approach is preferred.

Left and right heart catheterization

Radial access can be combined with upper limb percutaneous venous access to facilitate right and left heart catheterization. The procedure can be performed without withdrawal of systemic anticoagulation, since pressure haemostasis is safe and successful even in fully anticoagulated patients [27]. Our technique involves cleaning and draping the arm with an additional access area sited over the antecubital fossa. A tourniquet is placed over the upper arm beneath the drapes, and a suitable antecubital vein identified by palpation. Medial or lateral veins can be used if required. The vein is then punctured (we use a small syringe to aspirate blood through a conventional femoral puncture needle) and a guidewire inserted, followed by a short sheath. The tourniquet is then released and the sheath secured to the skin with intravenous cannula dressings. A conventional radial puncture is then performed to allow arterial access. A suitable right heart catheter can then be advanced up the arm over a guidewire.

For laterally positioned veins, a hydrophilic wire is usually necessary to navigate through the sharply angulated junction between the superficial and deep veins at the shoulder, but this can usually be easily accomplished under fluoroscopic control.

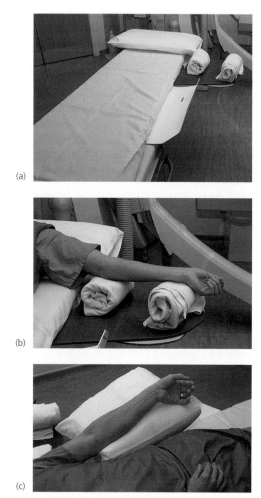

Figure 3.10 Left radial approach. (a) Setup; (b) puncture achieved with arm abducted; (c) arm brought to side for duration of case and lifted on a pillow.

Once the catheter enters the right atrium it is employed for the right heart study in a conventional fashion. At the end of the procedure, radial artery haemostasis is secured with a compression device. The venous sheath is removed and manual pressure applied for several minutes. If venous oozing continues after this, a tourniquet is applied over folded gauze squares, to apply prolonged pressure.

Image acquisition

Once a catheter has been positioned, radiographic image acquisition proceeds in a normal fashion. Over- and under-table shields should be positioned to reduce radiation exposure. Adducting the patient's arm allows the operator to stand further away from the radiation source. Attaching extension tubing between the end of the catheter and the manifold allows the operator to stand even further away. These measures ensure that radial operators are not exposed to excessive radiation. All conventional left- and right-sided views are easily obtained. Breath holding manoeuvres should be avoided as catheters inserted from the arm are highly sensitive to respiratory movement, and are therefore easily displaced. For lateral projections the image intensifier is taken below the normal horizontal position. This allows the X-ray beam to pass over the right arm lying alongside the thorax, producing a satisfactory lateral image.

Haemostasis

When image acquisition is complete, angiographic catheters are retrieved over a wire as described. The arterial sheath is then removed immediately and direct compression applied to the puncture site. Haemostasis can be achieved by either direct manual pressure or the use of a compression system. Application of direct manual pressure is time consuming, and therefore not generally employed. Older compression techniques used circumferential elastoplast dressings or a tourniquet to apply direct pressure. These systems are uncomfortable, produce venous stasis in the arm, and cannot be maintained in position for long time periods. We recommend the use of one of the many disposable unilateral compression systems. These systems are well tolerated and have a high success rate [28]. For example:

- The *RadiStop* consists of a back plate and compression pad. The wrist is secured in the support plate with an adjustable Velcro strap over the palm. A compression plate is supplied on a second Velcro strap. The compression plate is positioned over the puncture site and pressure applied whilst removing the sheath. The Velcro straps are then tightened and secured around the back plate to maintain compression (Figure 3.11). For routine diagnostic procedures we remove the RadiStop after 2 hours, placing a small elastoplast dressing over the puncture.

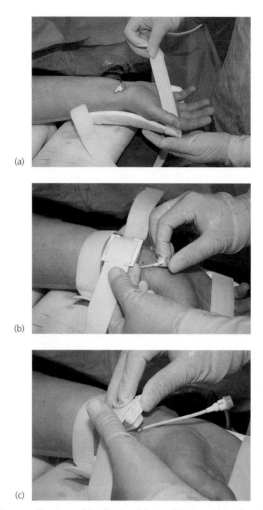

(a)

(b)

(c)

Figure 3.11   Application of RadiStop. (a) Application of backsplint;
(b) partial withdrawal of sheath and placement of compression pad;
(c) haemostatic pressure and complete sheath withdrawal.

- The *TR band* consists of an inflatable compression pad within a
  transparent wrist band. The compression pad is positioned over the
  puncture site and the band is wrapped around the wrist. The compression pad is then inflated with 15–18 mL of air and the sheath is
  removed (Figure 3.12). As with the RadiStop the device is deflated
  and removed after 2 hours, and an elastoplast dressing is applied.

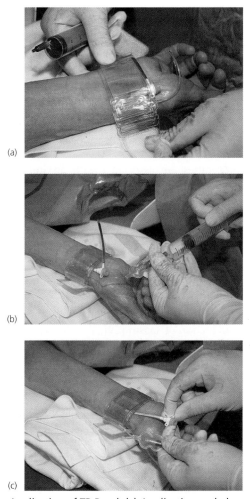

(a)

(b)

(c)

Figure 3.12 Application of TR Band. (a) Application and placement of TR Band; (b) partial withdrawal of sheath and partial inflation; (c) simultaneous cuff inflation and sheath withdrawal.

We use both of these highly effective devices in our unit. They both provide unilateral compression to the puncture site. The medial border of the wrist is free of compression, allowing unhindered venous drainage and ulnar arterial perfusion. Because of this, both devices are very well tolerated. The RadiStop is preferable for individuals with large wrists, the TR band for individuals with small wrists. For most patients the devices seem to be equivalent in efficacy. If bleeding continues after the initial compression period, the device is reapplied, and compression maintained until haemostasis is secure. For fully anticoagulated patients this may take several hours.

Complications and problem solving

The learning curve

Transradial procedures are associated with an important learning curve. The skills required to perform percutaneous femoral and radial procedures are identical. These skills require some adjustment and modification to facilitate the successful performance of a transradial procedure. Compared with the femoral artery, the radial artery is small and prone to spasm. Anatomical variations in the arm or head and neck vessels are less familiar to femoral operators. Catheter manipulation and optimization techniques require modification for radial operators. Studies suggest that the early failure rate for inexperienced operators will be around 10 per cent in the first 100 patients, usually due to puncture failure or induction of spasm [29]. This initial failure rate will be even higher if the operator has no previous experience of arm procedures. For experienced radial operators, procedure duration, radiation exposure and access failure rates are equivalent to those reported for femoral operators [14,15].

Before commencing a radial programme, femoral operators should get some hands-on training from an experienced radial operator. Education of other members of the catheterization laboratory team helps to promote a supportive atmosphere during the learning curve, when screening and procedural times will be prolonged, and access failure rate increased compared to routine femoral access [29]. It is wise to allow extra time for learning curve radial procedures when planning a list. Selection of suitable learning curve patients will help to minimize initial difficulties. Patients who have a radial artery that is difficult to palpate (often small, elderly or diabetic patients) are more difficult to cannulate. Very anxious individuals (particularly young patients) are prone to spasm and vasovagal reactions. Patients with extensive peripheral vascular disease or a large anteroposterior thoracic diameter are likely to have tortuous atheromatous vessels or an unfolded aorta, which will increase procedural complexity. These patients should be avoided during the learning curve in favour of individuals with easily palpable pulses and a normal body habitus.

For experienced operators, complications are very rare. These complications (including haematomas, arteriovenous fistulas, perforations and pseudoaneurysms) can usually be dealt with by local compression, and surgical intervention or the need for blood transfusion is exceedingly rare [30].

Puncture failure

As previously stated, this is predominantly a learning curve issue. When initial attempts to puncture the radial artery fail, it is recommended that the needle is withdrawn and direct pressure applied to the radial artery. This minimizes the risk of haematoma formation. Further attempts to puncture the artery may be successful if a more proximal site is selected (after administration of additional local anaesthetic). Repeated failed puncture attempts are often painful for the patient, and are likely to induce spasm or a vasovagal reaction.

During the learning curve puncture failure is inevitable, and operators should set a time limit for attempted puncture, defaulting to femoral access when they exceed their pre-set limit.

Coronary cannulation failure

After successfully positioning a radial sheath, operators can still encounter difficulties in cannulating the coronary arteries. Difficulties in advancing a guidewire up the arm or into the ascending aorta are usually related to anatomical issues in the arm or head and neck vessels. In this situation the wire should be withdrawn and an angiogram of the vessels obtained by contrast injection through the radial sheath in order to assess the anatomical configuration and decide on management [31]. The use of hydrophilic guidewires, steerable angioplasty wires and deep inspiration manoeuvres allow most of the difficulties to be overcome with experience.

Arterial spasm

Spasm can occur in the radial or brachial artery, and causes pain associated with equipment manipulation. Spasm is often precipitated by a painful or difficult radial artery puncture, and is therefore predominantly a learning curve issue. Preferentially selecting patients for easy punctures, using a vasodilator cocktail containing a calcium antagonist and nitrate, employing a long hydrophilic sheath and 5F catheters will limit the risk of spasm. When spasm is initiated by radial puncture it may be impossible to introduce a sheath, and the procedure may need to be completed via an alternative access site. Spasm that occurs in the upper arm with catheter exchanges indicates that an aberrant radial artery may be present. Administration of intra-arterial calcium antagonist and nitrates and downsizing the catheter calibre may allow the procedure to be completed. Brachial spasm during catheter exchanges can occur in small individuals, and usually responds to the above measures.

In rare instances, particularly if large-calibre non-hydrophilic sheaths are employed, sheath removal at the end of the procedure may be difficult because of diffuse intense radial spasm. In this situation it is important to avoid attempts at forceful sheath removal. This will cause more severe pain with aggravation of the spasm, or result in avulsion of the radial artery with severe bleeding into the forearm. We recommend the administration of small doses of intravenous diamorphine and a benzodiazepine for pain relief and sedation, along with intra-arterial calcium antagonists and nitrates administered through the sheath. A warm compress should be applied to the arm. After 10–15 minutes the sheath can usually be safely withdrawn. If these measures fail, an axillary nerve block using local anaesthetic can be easily administered (usually by an anaesthetist) to relax the radial artery and facilitate sheath removal.

Vasovagal reactions

Simple or complex vasovagal reactions can be precipitated by difficult or painful radial puncture (and are therefore predominantly a learning curve issue). In most patients a painful puncture initiates bradycardia and hypotension. These should rapidly respond to large doses of intravenous atropine and rapid fluid infusion. Once the heart rate and blood pressure are stabilized, it is usually safe to continue with the procedure. During the learning curve vasovagal reactions can occur in 5–10 per cent of patients, and the operator and laboratory staff should be prepared to respond rapidly to any evidence of a developing vasovagal reaction.

In some patients cannulation of the radial artery results in unexpected inferior ST elevation that occurs prior to coronary cannulation. This can be very profound, and is alarming to the operator. This syndrome has been described in other catheterization procedures, and is not related to coronary trauma or embolism [32]. Vagal stimulation can increase coronary resistance, leading to a reduction in regional myocardial blood flow independent of heart rate. This reflex ST segment change syndrome responds to large doses of atropine but not to nitrate, suggesting that it is vagally mediated. When the ST segment changes have resolved, it is usually safe to continue with the procedures as the risk of a further vagally mediated adverse event is low.

Puncture site problems

Local radial puncture site problems are very rare, with an incidence of less than 1 per cent [30]. Local puncture site infection can occur, presenting several days after the procedure with developing erythema, induration, swelling and possible pus formation [14]. This usually responds rapidly to a course of oral antibiotics. Localized haematomas can occur if initial access has been difficult (requiring multiple punctures) or the haemostasis device has not been optimally applied. These usually present shortly after application of the haemostasis device, with the development of swelling and induration at the puncture site [30]. If the situation is not easily controlled by repositioning and reapplying the haemostasis device, local compression applied directly to the puncture site is required. The easiest way to achieve secure local compression is by positioning several folded gauze squares over the puncture site, secured in position with a tightly applied circumferential sticking plaster dressing. A tourniquet is then positioned over the dressing to increase local compression. The compression is maintained for 30 minutes (if tolerated) and the tourniquet is then removed. The elastoplast dressing is maintained in position for a total of 4 hours. If the initial period of tourniquet compression fails to secure haemostasis, it can be reapplied for further periods as required.

Other local complications such as arteriovenous fistula or pseudoaneurysm are extremely rare, with an incidence rate of 1/2000 [30]. Pseudoaneurysms present early after the procedure with a localized painful swelling at the puncture site. Arteriovenous fistulas present with pain, paraesthesia and oedema of the affected hand, which may be associated with a localized murmur of thrill. Pseudoaneurysms and fistulas require evaluation by ultrasound to confirm the diagnosis. Some will respond to prolonged local compression (which can be applied for up to 72 hours), but surgical repair will be required if this fails [30].

The rate of local radial puncture site complications can be affected by equipment selection. The coating applied to some very hydrophilic radial sheath systems is easily stripped off and deposited in the skin. This induces a local allergic reaction that increases the risk of a puncture site complication. Although these very hydrophilic sheath systems are user friendly (and therefore helpful during the learning curve) they should be avoided by experienced operators in the interests of reducing local complications.

Vascular injury

Trauma to the arm or head and neck arteries can occur during a radial procedure. This most commonly occurs in the forearm, usually associated with the use of hydrophilic wires to negotiate tortuous segments of radial artery. A puncture with contrast extravasation is usually identified by contrast injection during fluoroscopic wire manipulation. When a radial puncture is identified, the procedure should be abandoned, and the forearm closely observed. If there is evidence of a developing forearm haematoma, local compression is applied to the puncture site (with a compression dressing and tourniquet or blood pressure cuff) and the arm is elevated. Close observation of the forearm and hand is required in these patients. If the haematoma continues to expand or there is any evidence of neurovascular compromise in the hand a developing compartment syndrome is possible, and urgent vascular surgical review is required.

Puncture or dissection of the brachial, axillary, subclavian or brachiocephalic vessels is very rare [29,30]. Performing catheter exchanges in tortuous or diseased vessels will increase the risk of vessel trauma, and an exchange length wire maintained in the ascending aorta is recommended for these patients. If there is extreme tortuosity in the proximal vessels, operators should consider the use of an alternative access site to minimize the risk of vessel trauma.

Further reading

Hamon Martial and McFadden Eugène. *Trans-radial Approach for Cardiovascular Interventions.* ESM editions, 2003.

References

1. Berry C, Kelly J, Cobbe SM *et al.* Comparison of femoral bleeding complications after coronary angiography versus percutaneous coronary intervention. *Am J Cardiol* 2004; **94:** 361–363.

2. Montalescot G, Chevalier B, Dalby MC *et al.* Description of modern practices of percutaneous coronary intervention and identification of risk factors for adverse outcome in the French nationwide OPEN registry. *Heart (British Cardiac Society)* 2005; **91:** 89–90.

3. de Queiroz Fernandes Araujo JO, Veloso HH, Braga De Paiva JM *et al.* Efficacy and safety of abciximab on acute myocardial infarction treated with percutaneous coronary interventions: a meta-analysis of randomized, controlled trials. *Am Heart J* 2004; **148:** 937–943.

4. Dauerman HL, Prpic R, Andreou C *et al.* Angiographic and clinical outcomes after rescue coronary stenting. *Cathet Cardiovasc Intervent* 2000; **50:** 269–275.

5. Koreny M, Riedmuller E, Nikfardjam M *et al.* Arterial puncture closing devices compared with standard manual compression after cardiac catheterization: systematic review and meta-analysis. *JAMA* 2004; **291:** 350–357.

6. Adams DF, Fraser DB, Abrams HL. The complications of coronary arteriography. *Circulation* 1973; **48:** 609–618.

7. Sones FM, Jr. Complications of coronary arteriography and left heart catheterization. *Cleveland Clin Q* 1978; **45:** 21–23.

8. Walton J, Greenhalgh RM. Brachial artery damage following cardiac catheterization. When to re-explore. *Eur J Vasc Surg* 1990; **4:** 219–222.

9. Hammacher ER, Eikelboom BC, van Lier HJ *et al.* Brachial artery lesions after cardiac catheterization. *Eur J Vasc Surg* 1988; **2:** 145–149.

10. Hildick-Smith DJ, Khan ZI, Shapiro LM *et al.* Occasional-operator percutaneous brachial coronary angiography: first, do no arm. *Cathet Cardiovasc Intervent* 2002; **57:** 161–165.

11. Campeau L. Percutaneous radial artery approach for coronary angiography. *Cathet Cardiovasc Diag* 1989; **16:** 3–7.

12. Kiemeneij F, Laarman GJ, de ME. Transradial artery coronary angioplasty. *Am Heart J* 1995; **129:** 1–7.

13. Kiemeneij F, Laarman GJ. Transradial artery Palmaz-Schatz coronary stent implantation: results of a single-center feasibility study. *Am Heart J* 1995; **130:** 14–21.

14. Eccleshall SC, Banks M, Carroll R *et al.* Implementation of a diagnostic and interventional transradial programme: resource and organizational implications. *Heart (British Cardiac Society)* 2003; **89:** 561–562.

15. Agostoni P, Biondi-Zoccai GG, de Benedictis ML *et al.* Radial versus femoral approach for percutaneous coronary diagnostic and

interventional procedures; Systematic overview and meta-analysis of randomized trials. *J Am Coll Cardiol* 2004; **44:** 349–356.

16. Louvard Y, Lefevre T, Allain A *et al.* Coronary angiography through the radial or the femoral approach: The CARAFE study. *Cathet Cardiovasc Intervent* 2001; **52:** 181–187.

17. Yokoyama N, Takeshita S, Ochiai M *et al.* Anatomic variations of the radial artery in patients undergoing transradial coronary intervention. *Cathet Cardiovasc Intervent* 2000; **49:** 357–362.

18. Abhaichand RK, Louvard Y, Gobeil JF *et al.* The problem of arteria lusoria in right transradial coronary angiography and angioplasty. *Cathet Cardiovasc Intervent* 2001; **54:** 196–201.

19. Allen EV. *Am J Med Sci* 1929; **178:** 237–244.

20. Barbeau GR, Arsenault F, Dugas L *et al.* Evaluation of the ulnopalmar arterial arches with pulse oximetry and plethysmography: comparison with the Allen's test in 1010 patients. *Am Heart J* 2004; **147:** 489–493.

21. Hosokawa K, Hata Y, Yano K *et al.* Results of the Allen test on 2,940 arms. *Ann Plast Surg* 1990; **24:** 149–151.

22. McGregor AD. The Allen test – an investigation of its accuracy by fluorescein angiography. *J Hand Surg Br Vol* 1987; **12:** 82–85.

23. Saito S, Ikei H, Hosokawa G *et al.* Influence of the ratio between radial artery inner diameter and sheath outer diameter on radial artery flow after transradial coronary intervention. *Cathet Cardiovasc Intervent* 1999; **46:**173–178.

24. Nagai S, Abe S, Sato T *et al.* Ultrasonic assessment of vascular complications in coronary angiography and angioplasty after transradial approach. *Am J Cardiol* 1999; **83:** 180–186.

25. Spaulding C, Lefevre T, Funck F *et al.* Left radial approach for coronary angiography: results of a prospective study. *Cathet Cardiovasc Diag* 1996; **39:** 365–370.

26. He GW. Verapamil plus nitroglycerin solution maximally preserves endothelial function of the radial artery: comparison with papaverine solution. *J Thorac Cardiovasc Surg* 1998; **115:** 1321–1327.

27. Hildick-Smith DJ, Walsh JT, Lowe MD *et al.* Coronary angiography in the fully anticoagulated patient: the transradial route is successful and safe. *Cathet Cardiovasc Intervent* 2003; **58:** 8–10.

28. Chatelain P, Arceo A, Rombaut E *et al.* New device for compression of the radial artery after diagnostic and interventional cardiac procedures. *Cathet Cardiovasc Diagn* 1997; **40:** 297–300.

29. Hildick-Smith DJ, Lowe MD, Walsh JT *et al.* Coronary angiography from the radial artery – experience, complications and limitations. *Int J Cardiol* 1998; **64:** 231–239.

30. Sanmartin M, Cuevas D, Goicolea J *et al.* Vascular complications associated with radial artery access for cardiac catheterization. *Rev Esp Cardiol* 2004; **57:** 581–584.

31. Esente P, Giambartolomei A, Simons AJ *et al.* Overcoming vascular anatomic challenges to cardiac catheterization by the radial artery approach: specific techniques to improve success. *Cathet Cardiovasc Intervent* 2002; **56:** 207–211.

32. Ludman PF, Hildick-Smith D, Harcombe A *et al.* Transient ST-segment changes associated with mitral valvuloplasty using the Inoue balloon. *Am J Cardiol* 1997; **79:** 1704–1705.

Percutaneous femoral approach

4

Recent decades have selected the femoral approach as the most widely practised access route for cardiac catheterization. The relative advantages of this as opposed to the radial or brachial approach are afforded by the size of the femoral artery, and general ease of accessing the vascular lumen from this point. The femoral vein, located immediately medial to the artery, is an ideal point for entry and execution of right heart catheterization and, where left and right studies are required simultaneously, the femoral route is an obvious first choice. The success of the technique is dependent upon adherence to a clearly defined procedural protocol. As with any approach, greater operator experience leads to greater ease in performing femoral route angiography, belying the potential pitfalls which exist.

As described elsewhere, there are relative contraindications to selecting the femoral approach. These include:

- Absent popliteal, dorsalis pedis or femoral pulses
- Extensive inguinal scarring
- Uncontrolled anticoagulation
- Abdominal aortic aneurysm
- Previous femoral vascular surgical grafting
- Inability of the patient to lie flat.

Some of these contraindications deserve qualification. Highly experienced operators might overcome the technical challenges imposed by any of the above and successfully carry out femoral route angiography. For example, the risk of iatrogenic trauma to an abdominal aneurysm might be circumvented by the careful use of an exchange length hydrophilic guidewire for the first pass and thereafter careful over-the-wire exchange of subsequent catheters. However with the appropriate skill base, the choice of an alternative route would avoid this risk altogether. Some texts indicate that femoral graft puncture is safe with appropriate care. It is our opinion that this should be avoided if possible, and an alternative route used if possible. The patient and vascular surgeon are unlikely to be grateful to the cardiologist for the graft occlusion which may ensue. Therefore while this chapter deals solely with the femoral approach, it is best for the cardiologist in training to become proficient in angiography via at least two access points. The novice should observe the contraindications detailed above.

Femoral anatomy and landmarks

The anatomy of the femoral region is illustrated in Figure 4.1a. The key landmarks for the operator are the inguinal ligament and the femoral head. A commonly recommended reference point is the inguinal skin crease, but this is unreliable as the position varies greatly between patients. In the obese subject the crease tends to lie inferior to the inguinal ligament. Thus palpable landmarks are preferable to visual ones. Both right- and left-sided femoral vessels may be selected for cannulation and the anatomical layout is mirrored on opposite sides. The

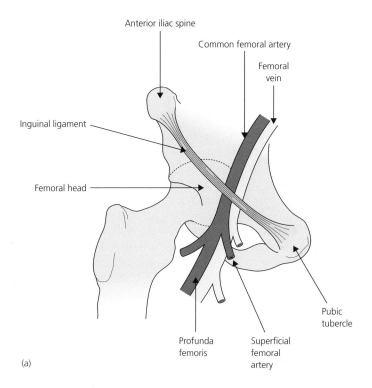

(a)

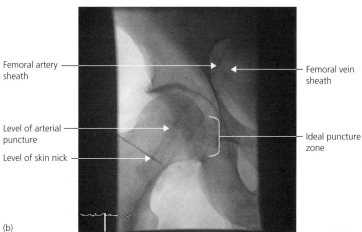

(b)

Figure 4.1 (a) Diagrammatic representation of femoral arterial anatomy. (b) Femoral arterial anatomy on X-ray.

inguinal ligament runs between the anterior superior iliac spine and the pubic tubercle. The point of reference for the operator is palpation of the common femoral artery by gentle compression against the femoral head. The femoral artery crosses posterior to the inguinal ligament at a point two-thirds along the ligament in a direction from iliac spine to pubis. The femoral vein is approximately 1 cm medial to the artery at the level of the inguinal ligament but passes posterior to the artery below this as it descends into the thigh. Anatomical variation occasionally locates the vein partially behind the artery at the level of the inguinal ligament. The femoral nerve is approximately 1 cm lateral to the artery.

It is important to understand the anatomy above and below the palpable segment of common femoral artery. The ideal point for cannulation is shown in Figure 4.1b. The main vessel bifurcates into the profunda femoris and the superficial femoral artery (SFA) 3–5 cm distal to the inguinal ligament. The bifurcation point is inferior to the femoral head as shown in Figure 4.1a. Therefore a 2–3 cm length of common femoral artery is palpable against the femoral head, representing the target for puncture (Figure 4.1b). Palpation of the vessel is augmented by asking the patient to laterally rotate the foot, thus bringing the vessels slightly anteriorly by movement of the femoral head. Puncturing too high or too low increases the risk of vascular complication. If the profunda, SFA, or the bifurcation point between these two is punctured, compression against the femoral head is not possible and haemostasis may prove difficult to achieve because only soft tissues lie posterior to this point. If the femoral vein, which runs posterior to the artery at this level, is punctured through the artery, arteriovenous fistula formation may ensue. Similarly, high penetration of the femoral artery, above the level of the inguinal ligament, may lead to local or retroperitoneal haemorrhage.

Percutaneous puncture of the femoral artery

The skin over the inguinal region is prepared with an appropriate antiseptic agent such as chlorhexidine or povidone iodine. Infiltration of the selected area with adequate amounts of local anaesthetic is essential; we normally use 10 mL of 1 per cent lignocaine (lidocaine), but some patients have required substantially more. If the right femoral route is selected, the operator's left index and middle fingers should be gently placed over the femoral artery at a point where the vessel is palpable against the femoral head. This acts as a reference point both for anaesthesia and for vessel cannulation. Thereafter 10–20 mL of 1 per cent or 2 per cent lignocaine (lidocaine) should be infiltrated using a 25 or 27 gauge needle, puncturing the skin 2 cm below the left index finger at an angle of approximately 45°.

Infiltration should incorporate superficial injection to anaesthetize the skin as well as deeper injection down to the level of the artery. The palpating left hand ensures that anaesthetic is deployed around and anterior to the planned puncture site. Clearly intra-arterial injection per se should be avoided and this may be checked by drawing back on the syringe plunger prior to deeper injection to ensure there is no flash-back of blood.

If combined arterial and venous cannulation is planned, infiltration of a similar amount of anaesthetic 1–2 cm medial to the first point is ideal at this stage of the procedure. There is some wisdom in allowing a dwell time of 2–3 minutes before any further action in order to allow the anaesthetic to take effect. The operator might be gainfully employed in other preparatory tasks at this stage.

A skin nick to a depth of 0.5 cm is made with a 10 or 11 scalpel blade over the infiltration point (care should be observed in the very thin patient as overzealous penetration with the blade might lacerate the artery). A small tunnel is then fashioned by blunt dissection with forceps. A modified Seldinger technique is employed. The original Seldinger technique advocated puncturing through both the anterior and posterior wall of the vessel with a hollow needle and drawing back. However a single clean puncture of the anterior wall assists haemostasis after the procedure and avoids bleeding from the back of the vessel while the procedure is taking place. The left hand is placed with index and middle fingers over the palpable segment of the common femoral artery. A bevelled cutting needle is introduced into the subcutaneous tunnel at an angle of 30–45° (Figure 4.2) with the bevel facing upwards (i.e. anteriorly in respect of the patient's anatomy) and advanced towards the palpating left hand.

The needle is held between index finger, middle finger and thumb of the right hand in the same fashion as a pen. Early operators used a pressure line to indicate penetration of the arterial lumen, but it is now more usual to have the back of the needle open to air to allow visualization of the arterial spurt. This simple visual reference may indicate the quality of the puncture as brisk arterial pulsation from the needle suggests that the distal end of the needle is ideally located within the common femoral artery lumen, poor flow suggests that an adjustment in position is required.

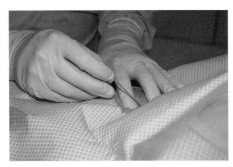

Figure 4.2 Puncture of right femoral artery by modified Seldinger technique.

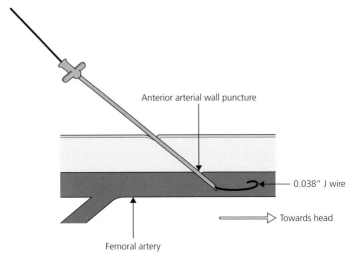

Figure 4.3 Correct needle position and wire advancement.

As soon as flow is seen, the needle is fixed by grasping the hub with the left hand and introducing a long or short 0.038″ J-tipped wire into the back of the needle and advancing (Figure 4.3). The wire should run smoothly if the distal needle is ideally situated. It is usual to feel a slight rasping of the wire against the anterior-facing bevel, but any significant resistance to the passage of the wire should alert the operator to stop. Firm spongy resistance often indicates that the wire is impacting on a vessel wall and if advanced may lead to a dissection of the arterial intima. If resistance does occur it is best to remove the wire from the needle, check that the arterial spurt is still present, adjust the position of the needle slightly to optimize this and then reintroduce the wire. If resistance has occurred it is often because the distal end of the needle is too deep and therefore close to the posterior vessel wall. A very small withdrawal may facilitate easy passage of the wire. Occasionally all that is required a slight rotation of the needle, to allow the bevel to be orientated towards the vessel lumen.

Once the wire has successfully passed into the artery for 10–15 cm, the needle is withdrawn and removed using the right hand while the left hand gently compresses the entry point to prevent back bleeding and haematoma formation.

The majority of centres conduct the angiographic procedure through a catheter sheath. For diagnostic purposes the most commonly selected sizes are 5, 6 or 7 French. Eight French systems are usually the domain of interventional procedures. The advantages of a smaller bore sheath and catheter include reduced time required in order to achieve haemostasis following the procedure, and a reduction in bleeding complications. This is offset against a slight reduction in torque with the smaller catheters and difficulty in attaining the same degree of opacification of the coronary arteries because of reduced contrast flow rates, often despite forcible injection.

The operator should select a sheath size consistent with the demands and complexity of each case. As shown in Figure 4.4, the preflushed haemostatic sheath and central introducer are passed over the wire. Entry through the skin and into the artery is achieved by firm pressure accompanied by gentle clockwise and anticlockwise rotational movements of the sheath. Once access is achieved, the left hand fixes the sheath in place and the right is used to simultaneously remove the wire and dilator. The sheath is then flushed through the side arm using heparinized saline.

Troubleshooting

Difficulty may be experienced if the patient has undergone a previous investigation via the same access route and scarring over the vessel means that the sheath does not pass easily. Use of force may buckle the sheath or damage the artery at the entry point. Under these circumstances it is best to predilate the tract with the introducer alone, and thereafter insert both sheath and introducer. Sometimes using the introducer from the sheath the size above will dilate a track; for example using a 7F dilator to create a track for a 6F sheath usually allows easy passage.

Occasionally, in spite of brisk arterial back flow being observed from the puncture needle, the J-shaped wire fails to advance easily. Adjustments

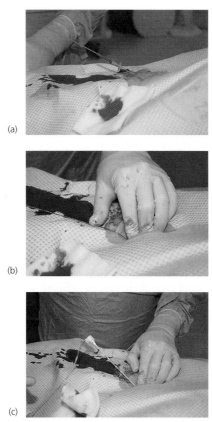

(a)

(b)

(c)

Figure 4.4   Insertion of a femoral arterial sheath. (a) Wire is introduced through needle. (b) Needle is removed and pressure applied over puncture site. (c) Sheath is advanced.

in position as described above usually resolve the problem. If not, a small injection of contrast into the back of the needle accompanied by fluoroscopy may delineate the anatomy, guiding further action. Hydrophilic wires should *not* be introduced into a cutting needle as inadvertent withdrawal of the wire may lead to it being severed by the cutting edge, resulting in loss of the distal wire into the vessel lumen. These wires should only be employed once the sheath, or at the very least the central introducer, are in the vessel.

If the iliac vessels are very tortuous, this may pose difficulty in rotating the diagnostic catheters once the procedure is underway. The problem may be circumvented by introducing a specifically designed longer sheath (approximately 25 cm) with reinforced radial strength which does not 'kink' in the tortuous segment. However, these can sometimes be a little inflexible and an additional trick is to pass the long sheath part way in to the artery so that the first part of the sheath is definitely within the true lumen of the artery. Then take the introducer out and pass a JR4 catheter, which can be steered/passed through a tortuous segment more easily than the stiff introducer. The sheath is then fully advanced over the top of the catheter.

Percutaneous puncture of the femoral vein

As described above, if venous access is sought then additional anaesthetic infiltration should be carried out medial to the arterial access point. Again it is important that lignocaine (lidocaine) is delivered both superficially and deeply. A further skin nick is made 1–2 cm medial to the arterial nick at the same level. Some operators prefer to undertake the venous puncture first but this is not essential. We recommend performing the venous puncture second, as the sheath within the artery provides a clearly palpable landmark. Fingers of the left hand press down firmly 2–3 cm above the venous skin nick to slow venous return and enhance distension of the vein. A 10 cm syringe containing 4–5 mL of heparinized saline is attached to the back of the needle and this is advanced at 45° cephalad. Once flashback of blood is achieved, the needle hub is steadied with the left hand and the syringe is gently removed. A J wire and sheath are introduced in the same manner as described for arterial cannulation.

In some patients the femoral vein may be in a posterior position relative to the artery at the level of the inguinal ligament. In such circumstances conventional puncturing in the manner described above may prove fruitless. A simple trick is to distract the artery a few centimetres laterally with sheath *in situ*, thus exposing the vein for a successful puncture. This is one reason for attaining the arterial access first.

Catheter selection

'All roads lead to Rome', or perhaps 'There are many ways to skin a cat' might be suitable proverbs to cover selective angiography of the coronary arteries and left ventricular angiography. For any chosen coronary ostium there are numerous diagnostic catheters which might be successfully manipulated into the opening for the purposes of imaging the anatomy. However, certain catheters are ideally suited to specific anatomical conditions. We describe the more commonly chosen options below.

The basic technique of catheter advancement from the femoral region involves an initial introduction of the catheter and 0.038′ 180 cm J wire into the sheath. Following this, the assistant or operator advances the wire for approximately 20 cm ahead of the catheter, ensuring unhindered passage. If any resistance is felt this should be announced and the advance of the wire should be stopped. Fluoroscopic screening at the level of the iliac vessels can alert the team to excessive tortuousity or stenoses, indicated by the wire doubling up and failing to progress. The catheter may be advanced gently along the fixed wire to the point of resistance, whereupon removal of the wire and imaging of a gentle injection of dye contrast will illustrate the anatomical difficulty.

The wire is advanced ahead of the catheter over the arch of the aorta. It should then be fixed in position with approximately 5 cm lying in the ascending aorta. The catheter may then be advanced over this to a suitable position near the relevant sinus of Valsalva (see below). Conventional teaching is that the ostium of the vessel is only engaged once the wire is removed and the catheter has been connected to the pressure transducer. Prior to this connection, operators are strongly advised to aspirate the open catheter end with a syringe until 5–10 mL of blood is obtained. This ensures that no air bubbles are retained in the catheter. Connection to the manifold is then carried out with saline running (a 'wet to wet' connection). The pressure line should then indicate a normal arterial trace, as covered elsewhere in this text.

Cannulation of coronary vessels

Left main coronary ostium

The most commonly selected catheter for the left coronary is the Judkins left with a 4 cm curve (JL4). In the vast majority of patients of normal stature and with no dilatation of the aortic root, this specifically designed catheter will easily engage the left main stem with minimal adjustment on the part of the operator. After passing over the arch

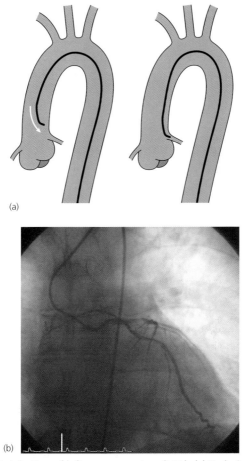

(a)

(b)

Figure 4.5   Intubation of left coronary artery (LCA). (a) Technique of intubation of LCA. (b) Correct position of JL4 catheter.

of the aorta the catheter tip is suspended just at the superior aspect of the left sinus of Valsalva (Figure 4.5). With the wire withdrawn and the system connected to pressure, the left main stem is engaged by gentle and controlled advancement of the catheter (Figure 4.5b). The ideal engagement is where the catheter tip is aligned with the main stem close

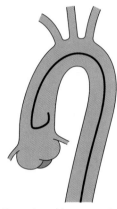

Figure 4.6   Enlarged aortic root and inappropriate catheter selection.

to horizontal on the fluoroscopy screen. This ensures that the subsequent dye injection attains optimal opacification with minimal risk of trauma to the intima from the jet.

In patients with an enlarged aortic root (typically those with long-standing hypertension or aortic valve disease) larger Judkins curves are required. If a JL4 is used there is a tendency for the catheter to 'wrap up' in the aortic root once the guidewire is withdrawn (Figure 4.6); in these cases JL4.5, 5 or 6 options are available for this purpose. The technique for engagement is the same as that for the smaller curve. In smaller subjects or in patients where the take-off of the left main stem is orientated more superiorly, smaller Judkins curves in the form of the JL3 or 3.5 are better suited to the task. Several angiographic projections suit engagement of the left main stem but perhaps the two best are straight posteroanterior (PA) and left anterior oblique (LAO) with caudal tilt (spider view). These views display the anatomy clearly and are helpful if difficulty is experienced with the JL4 in the first instance.

Anatomical variants can present a further challenge. One regular finding is that of separate origins of the left anterior descending (LAD) and circumflex vessels with no clear left main vessel. It is possible under most circumstances to cannulate both arteries individually with a JL4 (Figure 4.7). If the circumflex is selected on the first pass, cannulation of the LAD will be facilitated by removing the catheter tip from this, very slight anticlockwise rotation and re-advancing the catheter. However much time may be wasted in trying to achieve imaging of

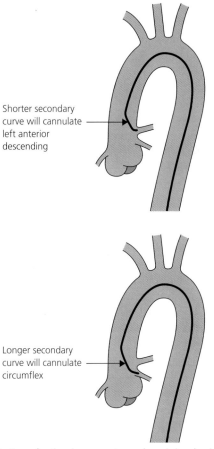

Shorter secondary
curve will cannulate
left anterior
descending

Longer secondary
curve will cannulate
circumflex

Figure 4.7   Catheter selection in separate and conjoined origins.

both vessels with this one catheter. A simpler option is to use two separate left Judkins models differing by 0.5 cm. The smaller of the two (e.g. JL3.5) will usually pass into the LAD and the larger (e.g. JL4) into the circumflex. Another common variant is where the ostium of the left main stem originates away from the usual position and is therefore not in line with the plane of the Judkins catheter design. Typically it originates more superiorly – closer to the sinotubular junction. Gentle manipulation of the JL4 with very slight anticlockwise rotation usually yields success.

If excessive manipulation of the catheter is required the Judkins left will repeatedly 'wrap up' in the aorta. A number of alternative catheters might be more suitable and the most commonly chosen option is the Amplatz range. These are also available is increasing sized curves from AL1 to 4, although it is uncommon to require larger than an AL2 for most anatomy. The method of introduction of the Amplatz catheter is slightly different to the Judkins.

The left Amplatz catheter is passed over the aortic root on the guidewire and introduced onto the left sinus of Valsalva with the tip initially pointing downward (Figure 4.8a). The wire is removed. Cannulation of the ostium of the left main stem is then achieved by advancing the catheter tip so that it rides up the wall of the sinus until it engages the vessel (Figure 4.8b). The engagement may then be optimized by either gentle retraction, gentle rotation, or by the patient inhaling deeply. Larger curves are suited to the more dilated aorta. Care needs to be exercised both on engagement and removal of this catheter, avoiding excessively deep cannulation and trauma to the vessel. Once the catheter is in place withdrawal may, paradoxically, engage the tip more deeply. Therefore once image acquisition is complete, by gently advancing and simultaneously rotating the Amplatz, the tip may easily disengage, allowing for withdrawal.

Right coronary artery

For imaging of the right coronary artery (RCA), vein grafts and internal mammary arteries, the operator should always remember that 'slower is faster'. Rushing the delicate rotation required during successful engagement often leads to a prolonged procedure and a tired, frustrated cardiologist. Therefore imaging these vessels should be regarded as a delicate art requiring deftness of touch.

The most commonly used catheter for the right coronary is the Judkins right with a 4 cm curve (JR4). As with the left coronary catheters, smaller and larger curve sizes are available to suit anatomical variation. If the take-off of the RCA is orientated superiorly, a JR3.5 may be more suitable and conversely the JR5 might be suitable for inferior take-off. However experienced operators can usually achieve success using the JR4 for most variants. The LAO projection is best for the procedure. As with the left, the catheter is introduced into the aortic root on the wire, but in this case it is advanced down to the level of the aortic valve and the wire is withdrawn. The JR4 will be orientated

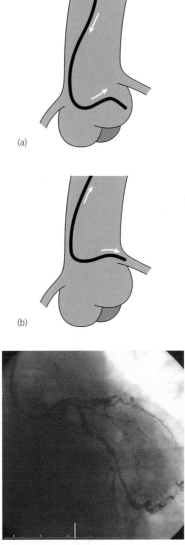

(a)

(b)

(c)

Figure 4.8 Correct manipulation of Amplatz catheter. (a) Advancing the Amplatz catheter will cause the tip to lift. (b) Traction will cause the catheter tip to advance and descend. (c) Left Amplatz catheter in the left coronary artery ostium.

towards the right hand side of the fluoroscopy screen at this time, pointing in the direction of the left coronary sinus (Figure 4.9a,b). The catheter, attached to pressure transducer, should be gently withdrawn to align the tip with the sinotubular junction and gentle rotation should follow. This may be either clockwise or anticlockwise but on both counts should take place slowly.

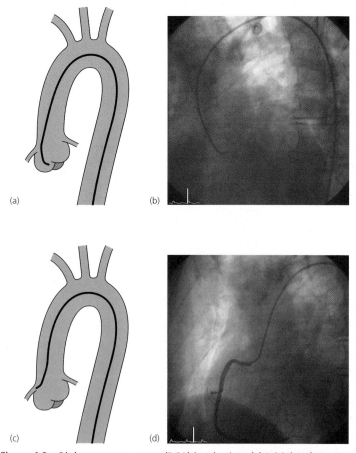

(a)

(b)

(c)

(d)

Figure 4.9   Right coronary artery (RCA) intubation. (a) Initial catheter position. (b) JR4 catheter approaching RCA ostium. (c) RCA intubation showing correct catheter position in the RCA ostium. (d) RCA injection.

Some torque will be stored in the catheter as it passes over the arch of the aorta so there is some wisdom is pausing occasionally and allowing the catheter to continue rotation alone, driven by this stored potential. With good fortune the catheter tip will be seen to move leftward and downward on the fluoroscopy screen as the RCA is engaged (Figure 4.9c,d).

Common mistakes include overzealous rotation of the catheter, with the inexperienced operator fruitlessly spinning the catheter tip somewhere above the aortic valve! Slower is faster. If the catheter tip is too low at the time of rotation it will tend to rotate freely through the right coronary sinus of Valsalva without engaging the coronary ostium, so it is important to begin the movement with the tip at, or above, the level of the sinotubular junction. Occasionally, over-rotation of the catheter leads to excessively deep engagement of the RCA and this is resolved by gentle counter-rotation and withdrawal.

It is very important to check the pressure tracing to exclude damping (ventricularization of the trace). This may be caused by spasm of the RCA, a true ostial stenosis or engagement of the conus branch. The RCA and conus branch do not respond favourably to prolonged damping. A *very* gentle injection of dye will delineate the position of the catheter tip. If it is in the conus branch, instant removal is recommended. (Firm injection of dye into the conus branch invariably leads to ventricular fibrillation.) If the tip is in the RCA, gentle withdrawal, possibly with intracoronary nitrate delivery, may resolve the damping. If the damping persists the catheter should be removed and gentle re-engagement carried out.

The problem of rotation using the Judkins right may be circumvented by using a catheter with preshaped orientation toward the right coronary sinus. The Williams catheter fulfils this requirement and, some may argue, is a suitable first line choice for imaging the RCA. The angulation of the primary curve is close to 90°. As the catheter passes over the arch of the aorta and down to the level of the valve it is orientated towards the RCA and very often engages on the first pass. Thus it is best to halt the progression of the catheter above the level of the sinotubular junction, remove the wire, and gently advance on pressure without rotating initially. Gentle rotation may be required if engagement is not immediately successful.

Occasionally the right coronary ostium is high and anterior and even above the sinotubular junction. Under these circumstances right Amplatz or even left Amplatz catheters are suited to locating the origin, achieved by gentle rotation and test injections of small aliquots of contrast in order to guide efforts. Using both LAO and RAO projections further assist identification of the site of the ostium, looking in particular for an anterior take-off.

Cannulation of saphenous vein grafts

Coronary bypass surgery has been performed over the past three decades and it is not unusual for patients to require further angiographic study in the years following this procedure. Some operations have been remarkably successful at stabilizing symptoms over more than a decade and therefore some of the graft restudies explore postoperative anatomy relating to surgery in the late 1980s or early 1990s. Core knowledge of surgical techniques and their evolution over this time scale may assist the angiographer in successfully identifying the relevant grafts. Furthermore, locating the original operation record is invaluable.

The historically recommended strategy of beginning a search for saphenous vein grafts with an aortagram is no longer appropriate. This should be employed as a last resort where one is unable to identify grafts by the means described below. Conventionally, grafts supplying left coronary vessels arise from the left anterior aspect of the aorta, while those supplying the right arise from the right anterior aspect. Of the left coronary grafts, those feeding the circumflex territory are usually placed more superior to those supplying the LAD or diagonals. Any variation, such as a posterior aortic origin, is usually indicated in the operative record, reinforcing the importance of securing this prior to embarking on the procedure.

It is sensible to begin the search for grafts using the correct catheter! The left coronary bypass and right coronary bypass catheters are, as suggested by the names, specifically designed for their purpose and are an ideal first line choice.

In the RAO projection the left anterior aspect of the aorta is represented by the right silhouetted border of the aorta on the imaging screen. The left coronary grafts usually arise at varying points of elevation above the sinus of Valsalva along this border. Therefore by gently turning the left coronary bypass catheter so as to orientate the tip towards this border, the graft origins may be located by simply 'trawling' up and down this surface. Locating the graft, or stump remnant of the graft, is indicated by the catheter tip catching and the point appears

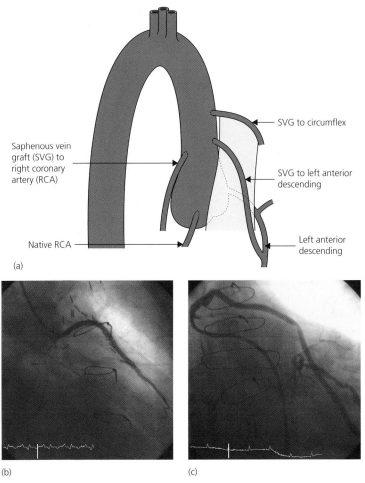

(a)

(b)   (c)

Figure 4.10 (a) Graft location (right anterior oblique view). (b) Injection of saphenous vein graft to left anterior descending. (c) Injection of saphenous vein graft to circumflex.

fixed while the rest of the catheter oscillates with systolic flow in the aorta (Figure 4.10a–c). A gentle test injection confirms position. Each graft should be imaged in at least two views, and images of stumps should also be acquired to confirm any graft occlusion. A graft which has not been identified should not be presumed to be occluded.

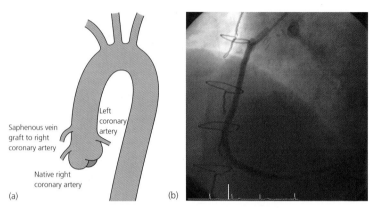

Figure 4.11   Orientation of ostium for saphenous vein graft to right coronary artery (RCA) (left anterior oblique view). (b) RCA graft injection.

Alternative catheter options for locating the left-sided coronary grafts include the Judkins right 4 and the left Amplatz 1 or 2.

The right coronary vein graft is best located using the LAO projection. Again the silhouette of the ascending aorta acts as a guide. The usual site of the graft origin is on the left aspect of the aorta (as seen on the screen in this view) at the point of maximal lateral convexity (Figure 4.11a,b). The right coronary bypass catheter has a more open primary curve than the JR4 and is ideal for locating and opacifying the graft. Occasionally the take-off of the graft is oriented more vertically and under these conditions a multipurpose catheter may give good engagement and excellent opacification. Adequate opacification is important in imaging of all grafts, because the large calibre of these conduits tends to predispose to streaming of dye if injection rates are too slow. The correct catheter should be favourably aligned with the proximal graft and this enhances the opacification – the wrong catheter choice will lead to suboptimal pictures.

Cannulation of left and right internal mammary arterial grafts

Arterial conduits were first employed for coronary bypass surgery almost four decades ago. The most commonly used of these is the left internal mammary artery (LIMA), which exhibits excellent long-term patency rates. Somewhat more recently the right-sided equivalent (RIMA) has been successfully used to graft both right- and left-sided coronary arteries. A sound knowledge of the anatomy of vessels originating from the aortic arch, as well as the subclavian system and branches, is essential before attempting to cannulate the internal mammary arteries.

The LIMA arises from the left subclavian vessel just distal to, and on the contralateral side to, the origin of the left vertebral artery (as shown in Figure 4.12a). The thyrocervical trunk arises close to the LIMA origin and is often engaged in the process of seeking the graft. The left

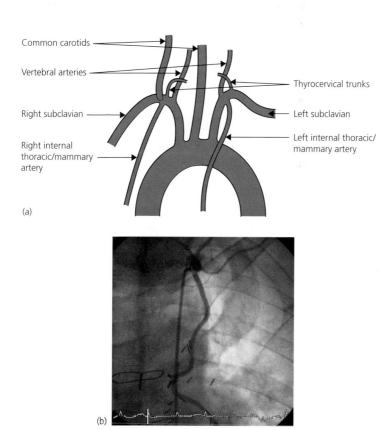

Figure 4.12   (a) Origin of internal mammary arteries. (b) Left internal mammary artery catheter (LIMA) *in situ* and selective LIMA injection.

carotid has a separate origin to the subclavian on this side. On the right side the right inominate artery divides into the right carotid and the right subclavian. The RIMA origin is again distal and contralateral to the vertebral artery. Clearly, unnecessary cannulation of the head and neck vessels is best avoided during the search for the LIMA or RIMA. The principle of 'slower is faster' prevails in this situation as much as in the cannulation of native coronaries.

For both grafts the appropriately named internal mammary artery (IMA) catheter is the best choice. This has a fairly tight primary curve, allowing for full engagement of the ostium of the vessel. The PA projection is best for cannulation.

In order to locate the LIMA the catheter should be advanced to the aortic arch on the J wire and the wire should be withdrawn slightly in order to give the tip greater flexibility. At this point the convex part of the primary and secondary curve is pressed against the superior aspect of the aortic arch slightly proximal to the left subclavian origin. By simultaneously maintaining this gentle pressure on the arch and rotating the catheter tip slowly in a counterclockwise direction, the tip should enter the subclavian vessel. This manoeuvre may be aided by asking the patient to place the left arm above his or her head.

An alternative technique is to approach the aortic arch in the LAO 50° view. In many subjects the origin of the left subclavian is superimposed on the right-hand border of the trachea, as seen by the operator on the viewing screen in this view. The catheter is advanced beyond the origin over the J wire, and the wire then withdrawn back into the catheter. With gentle traction and counterclockwise rotation the catheter will often enter the subclavian artery.

The J wire is then advanced over the first curve of the subclavian and the catheter is then advanced to a position beyond the LIMA origin and the wire removed. Test injections of dye tend to produced a warm sensation in the arm or possibly head and neck and the patient should be forewarned of this. By gently withdrawing the catheter to the apex of the subclavian, a test of dye will usually indicate the location of the LIMA ostium. The catheter tip should be positioned just distal to this and rotated very slowly counterclockwise, bringing it to a more anterior orientation. This should lead to engagement of the LIMA. Severe tortuosity of the subclavian vessel can lead to difficulty in this phase of the procedure. Perseverance and a slow gentle approach usually reap rewards. If unsuccessful, a non-selective injection of the LIMA may suffice. The opacification of the graft may be enhanced by inflating a blood pressure cuff above systolic pressure on the left arm at the time of injection, thus preventing dye flow in the arm. If there is difficulty, the left radial offers an alternative approach, where cannulation of the LIMA is often very simple.

The manoeuvre for locating the RIMA is similar. The catheter is placed in the arch just proximal to the innominate origin and the same simultaneous pressure plus rotation leads to the tip of the catheter entering this vessel. At this point a test injection will delineate the take-off of the right carotid and subclavian respectively. Gentle rotation of the catheter will orientate the tip more favourably toward the sub-clavian and the wire is advanced into it. Once this is achieved the distal end of the catheter should be deployed beyond the RIMA origin. With the wire removed the catheter tip should point inferiorly and anteriorly (achieved by very slight clockwise rotation). Gentle withdrawal often leads to a good engagement of the vessel. As with the LIMA, anatomical variation may lead to this being a taxing procedure.

Both the LIMA and RIMA have low incidence of atherosclerosis. Therefore once engaged, a single dynamically panned acquisition of the opacified graft connecting to the coronary vessel in the PA projection is usually sufficient to determine the status of the graft itself. However a further two or even three acquisitions in different projections of the graft anastamosis and distal native vessel bed will provide important supplementary information. This is the usual site for lesion development. Therefore it is not necessary to begin these latter imaging sequences superiorly in the neck at the catheter tip, but rather it is better to focus on the heart. In the process of locating the origin of these two grafts, great care should be taken not to traumatize the vessels, as dissection of the IMA or subclavian may ensue, often with dramatic and unwanted consequences.

Other arterial grafts

It is unusual to encounter conduits other than those described above. However, in an effort to carry out total arterial revascularization of the heart other vessels such as the radial artery and gastroepiploic artery have been used in some patients. The radial artery is harvested from the arm and is either connected in a similar site and fashion to saphenous vein grafts with the superior origin in the ascending aorta, or alternatively it is connected to the descending aorta. Once again the importance

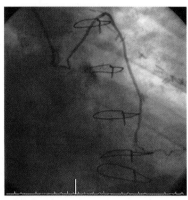

Figure 4.13   Injection of radial artery graft showing typical features of small calibre – the string sign.

of obtaining the operation note is emphasized. Cannulation of the radial graft in the usual site originating from the ascending aorta is very similar to the procedure described with respect to vein grafts. The vessel is remarkably prone to spasm and the images obtained on cannulation are often somewhat underwhelming (the 'string sign') (Figure 4.13). If the radial graft is of small calibre, then a gentle introduction of intra-coronary nitrate may be necessary to exclude catheter-induced spasm.

The right gastroepiploic may be freed from its usual course supplying stomach and diverted superiorly to connect to coronary vessels supplying the inferior wall of the heart, such as the posterior descending artery. The gastroepiploic artery is engaged by the use of catheters designed to cannulate the coeliac trunk and manipulation of these catheters, hydrophilic wires, and low profile probing catheters to pass through the common hepatic, gastroduodenal and gastroepiploic vessels respectively. The procedure is often challenging and represents unfamiliar territory for most cardiologists. Moreover these cases are uncommon. Therefore there is some wisdom in seeking help from colleagues in vascular radiology when carrying out this procedure.

Haemostasis

An important determinant of successful haemostasis is successful puncture in the first instance. By observing important principles such as correct anatomical positioning and only a single anterior pass into the femoral artery, haemostasis can be simplified and complications minimized. A number of groin closure devices are now available but simple digital compression remains the first choice for most units.

Digital technique

It is important for the staff removing the femoral sheath to have the same understanding of the anatomy and puncture procedure as the operator (understanding that it is not always the operator carrying out haemostasis). Distal pulses are checked prior to sheath removal. Because the cutting needle was directed at an angle of 30–45° cephalad when entering the femoral artery, the cutaneous landmark of vessel entry is usually 0.5–1 cm superior to the skin nick. With the patient lying recumbent with arms at the side, the middle three fingers of the operator's left hand are used to apply firm pressure above and on this vessel entry point. Simultaneously the vascular sheath is withdrawn with the right hand and firm downward pressure is applied with the left to achieve haemostasis. The skin nick should remain visible just below the index finger of the left hand at all times as this gives an indication of the progress of the procedure and allows for detection of any bleeding due to malpositioning. Gentle swabbing of the skin nick is helpful but the area in question should not be concealed by a swab during this process as it will impair the identification of a haematoma.

Firm, but not brutal, pressure is required. The operator should be able to detect the femoral pulsation beneath the fingers of the left hand. Complete occlusion of the femoral artery is *not* a prerequisite for success, and there is evidence to support that haemostasis is better and more quickly achieved if antegrade flow is maintained. Digital control over the puncture site with retained flow within the femoral vessel allows for delivery of clotting factors and platelets to the point. If pressure assistance is required, simply placing the fingers of the right hand over the left will usually suffice. The use of a fist or elbow is not only excessive, but often results in poor location of the puncture site and a resultant haematoma. Another common mistake is to carry out digital compression too low, thus failing to control the bleeding point, with similar consequences.

Firm pressure should be maintained for 5 minutes, and lighter pressure should then continue for a further 5–10 minutes. The longer this phase of haemostasis is carried out the better the outcome. Longer compression times are advocated for a total of 20 minutes for patients with hypertension, marked obesity, calcified femoral vessels or those with a wide pulse pressure such as in severe aortic incompetence. Once the operator has completed the compression, the fingers are removed from the site and the patient is asked to cough gently while the area is observed. Distal pulses are palpated and recorded and the groin is examined for either ooze or subcutaneous haematoma formation. If no rebleeding ensues, the patient is advised to remain recumbent with head relaxed on the pillow (in order to prevent muscular distraction of inguinal area by lifting the head) and this position should be maintained for approximately 1 hour. Over the subsequent 2-hour period the patient is brought gradually to a 45° upright angle on the recovery trolley and allowed to mobilize within the ward or unit.

Important consideration must be given to anticoagulation. If intraprocedural heparin has been administered sheath removal should be delayed until the activated clotting time (ACT) has fallen to 150 seconds or less. If there is any delay between the procedure and sheath removal, further local anaesthetic should be administered to the site in advance as the initial effects will have worn off. Prophylactic administration of 600 mg of atropine is advised. Poor anaesthesia will not only result in an unpleasant experience for the patient but will also greatly increase the likelihood of a vasovagal reaction when compression begins. If larger gauge sheaths have been used or concomitant agents such as glycoprotein IIb/IIIa antagonists are administered, prolonged compression is advised. This may be facilitated by the use of mechanical devices following the digital procedure (e.g. Femostop; USCI, Billerica, MA, USA) which then free the staff for other tasks.

If a left and right heart study has been performed, femoral venous sheath removal should follow the removal of the arterial sheath by 5–10 minutes, once the lighter compression phase is underway and control of the arterial puncture site is well established. This is achieved by simply moving the three fingers of the operator's left hand forward (medial to the arterial site) in order to simultaneously maintain pressure over the arterial puncture with the mid portion of the fingers, while the fingertips are applied over the venous puncture point. The sheath is removed with the right hand and modest pressure maintained over the whole region for a further 10 minutes.

In a busy unit, high throughput or a lack of operator patience may lead to inadequate time for digital compression. This becomes a false economy if further time needs to be invested to deal with problems such as late rebleeding or haematoma formation. Provided some arterial flow is maintained, digital compression of the femoral artery may be continued for a prolonged period without any ill effect. Observation of a general rule of 'longer is better' will prevent many bleeding complications, especially for the novice.

Closure devices

Early versions of groin closure devices were disadvantaged by fairly high failure rates and high incidence of complications. As a result of this the design in a number of these devices has been refined by the respective manufacturers and they now offer a useful haemostasis option in the catheter laboratory. As with any other aspect of angiography, the success of closure is influenced by the skill and experience of the operator.

Angio-Seal

Several devices employ a collagen plug in order to facilitate the patient's intrinsic haemostatic mechanisms. The Angio-Seal (St Jude Medical) comprises three absorbable components, namely a suture, an anchor and the collagen plug. The anchor is delivered into the lumen through a designated sheath and is then withdrawn on the suture to abut against the intima of the artery. The plug is then pushed down into the skin track at the same time as a the suture tightens and knots (STS platform). The suture is then trimmed at skin level. The device is useful in patients on anticoagulation or those with difficulty in lying recumbent following angiography. A femoral angiogram through the angiography sheath is advocated before using this device. This ensures that the original puncture is into the common femoral artery. If it is not, the closure device should not be used. Other contraindications include significant peripheral vascular disease involving the iliac and femoral vessels, excessive tortuosity, or previous vascular site complications. These contraindications are applicable to most of the other devices described below.

Vasoseal

Like the Angio-Seal, the Vasoseal (Datascope) is based on a collagen plug. An arteriotomy locator is inserted at the time of removal of the procedure sheath in order to determine the depth of the vessel puncture beneath the skin. Using the markers on the locator a collagen cartridge is delivered into the skin track by pressing on a plunger and removing the delivery sheath. No suture is involved in the mechanism. A short period of firm pressure is required after delivery to achieve haemostasis.

Perclose

The Perclose (Abbott Vascular) employs a different principle. It relies on the successful 'suturing' of the margins of the arteriotomy site by passing fine nitonal needles through the vessel wall. It requires some dexterity on the part of the operator and is usually best conducted with an active assistant. The more refined Proglide version has a pre-tied knot, which is more easily delivered than previously. Once the suture is engaged within the arterial wall the knot is pushed to closure with a designated probe and the suture is trimmed.

Starclose

Again a different principle is engaged. The Starclose (Abbott Vascular) system involves the accurate location of the vessel wall through a delivery sheath. Once achieved, a petal-shaped nitonal clip is delivered to the external aspect of the vessel. Closure is achieved by the clip grasping and sealing the external edges of the puncture point. The clip remains in place indefinitely.

Groin complications

As described elsewhere in this text there are a number of serious, but fortunately rare, complications which may arise from cardiac catheterization via any route. This section is devoted to those that are specific to the femoral route.

Bleeding

As mentioned above, if care and attention are paid to both the correct puncture technique and fastidious haemostasis, bleeding complications can be minimized. The advent of smaller gauge sheaths and catheters has significantly reduced this type of complication when compared to previous decades.

Minor regional bruising is common following a diagnostic procedure via the femoral route. It may not be apparent on the day of the procedure, but rather becomes more pronounced in subsequent days. It is self-limiting and usually only of cosmetic relevance to the patient.

Haematoma formation is more concerning. The size of the collection may range from a few centimetres in diameter to a grapefruit-sized haematoma which rapidly accrues, causing haemodynamic embarrassment, requiring urgent transfusion and an urgent vascular surgical opinion. Predisposing factors contributing to bleeding risk include increased age, either marked obesity or extreme thinness, hypertension, tortuous calcified femoral vessels, anticoagulation, or wide pulse pressure in conditions such as aortic incompetence. All of the technical issues related to puncture site are of prime importance (see above). If the haematoma develops during the course of the procedure, it may be related either to traumatic entry through the vessel wall or to a puncture of the posterior wall which is not sealed by the sheath *in situ*. One simple manoeuvre is to up-size the sheath as this may stem the flow from the anterior puncture. Alternatively manual compression until the case is complete will usually stem the progression of the bleeding. Continued compression in transferring the patient to the recovery zone (or even sheath removal within the catheter lab) is advisable. It is important to note that the earlier a haematoma is compressed, the easier it is to control.

If a modest or large haematoma develops while the patient is in the recovery area, compression is once again the mainstay of treatment. This complication may be evident just before, during or a considerable time after the scheduled sheath removal (late rebleed). Therefore the recovery area protocol must promote vigilance for this problem. Compression over the puncture site is achieved by firm digital pressure, while more diffuse pressure is applied to the rest of the haematoma area with a flat hand or perhaps aid such as a sandbag. The first sign of success is where the initially hard, rubbery collection of blood in the soft issue of the upper leg softens. It is sensible to send a blood sample for cross-match and set up a colloid infusion in the interim. It is also important to administer parenteral analgesia as the process is often very painful for the patient. In very severe cases a surgical opinion should be sought. Even if the bleeding is successfully resolved, it is advisable to admit the patient to an overnight bed from the day case facility for observation.

Occasionally the bleeding problem may be more covert. If the groin puncture is above the inguinal ligament it is not possible to adequately compress the entry site and blood may track into the retroperitoneal space. This presents as unexplained hypotension following the procedure and may be accompanied by ipsilateral loin pain. Fluid resuscitation and/or transfusion should be backed up by imaging confirmation via ultrasound or computerized tomography. It is unusual for this complication to require surgical correction.

If a connection remains between the femoral artery puncture site and a haematoma, creating a fluid core, a false aneurysm develops. By virtue of its name the aneurysm has no true wall and is therefore at risk of rupture. Clinical signs to suggest that a groin swelling is not simply a clot include a pulsatile nature (best assessed by fingers on either side rather than above the aneurysm because femoral artery pulsation may simply be transmitted through an overlying haematoma) or the presence of a bruit. Confirmation of the diagnosis is by ultrasound and this will identify the size and position of the neck. The helpful ultrasonographer may be able to compress this point with the probe for 20–30 minutes and then reassess the flow. Alternatively a procoagulant may be injected into the aneurysm while the neck is occluded with the probe. If neither of these measures prove successful, surgical correction may be required for the persistent case.

An alternative route for blood from femoral puncture to track is into an adjacent vein, if this too was punctured during the study. This leads to the late formation of an arteriovenous fistula, identified clinically by a continuous humming bruit. Surgical correction is often required. Both this and pseudoaneurysm formation are more likely if the puncture is too low, and in particular at the point where the superficial femoral artery and profunda diverge.

Dissection

Traumatic iatrogenic dissection of the common femoral vessel is usually induced by rough handling of the artery with either sheath, catheter or guidewire. By simply employing a cautious approach of never advancing equipment where spongy resistance is encountered, the complication may be minimized. If a dissection is suspected during the course of the procedure it may be confirmed by dye injection with a digital acquisition (Figure 4.14). As in most cases the elevated intimal flap is against the direction of arterial flow, the majority of limited

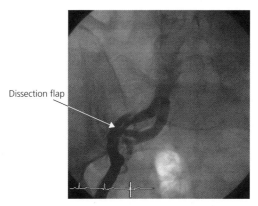

Figure 4.14 Iliac artery dissection.

dissections will settle spontaneously if they are not aggravated by further trauma. An experienced operator may circumvent the dissection site by careful negotiation with a hydrophilic wire under fluoroscopic guidance, thus completing the case. The novice is advised to seek assistance or choose an alternative access route if a dissection is seen. Rarely a spiralling dissection may result from catheter or wire trauma, compromising flow to the leg, and this requires an urgent surgical opinion.

Thrombosis and embolism

Fortunately, femoral arterial thrombosis is now very rare. This is largely due to the down-sizing of equipment thus maintaining arterial flow past the sheath during the course of the procedure. Predisposing factors to thrombosis include peripheral vascular disease and prolonged sheath dwell time. If a sheath is left *in situ* on return to recovery or a ward, the lumen should be flushed with heparinized saline and patency maintained with a pressure line attached to the side arm. This will also prevent inadvertent distal seeding of clot if the sheath is then flushed either for exchange or reuse for a subsequent procedure.

If either arterial thrombosis or embolism occur they are accompanied by the all of the signs of distal limb ischaemia. An early surgical opinion should be sought if any of the following are present:

- Pain
- Diminished pulses
- Prolonged capillary filling time
- Pale cold leg.

Conservative measures such as anticoagulation and the administration of vasodilators such as prostacyclins will often suffice for the milder cases. In the more severe cases embolectomy may be required. Femoral venous thrombosis and subsequent pulmonary embolism is also rare. In a similar fashion prolonged dwell time for a venous sheath will increase the risk of this problem. If a large femoral haematoma has formed, the compression effect may impede venous flow and also predispose to this problem. The incidence of this complication is largely averted by appropriate sheath management as described above.

Further reading

Baim Donald S and Grossman William (eds). *Grossman's Cardiac Catheterization, Angiography, and Intervention*, 6th edn. Philadelphia: Lippincott Williams & Wilkins, 2000.

Kern MJ (ed.) *Cardiac Catheterization Handbook*, 2nd edn. St Louis: Mosby, 1995.

Catheterization: techniques and interpretation 5

Setting up

Every centre will set up trolleys and the patients differently. Some centres do not utilize radiographers in the room, and the cardiologist has to set up each shot, cone down with the image intensifier shields and pan to follow the image on the viewing screen, whilst a scrub nurse injects. Others have a radiographer and no scrub nurse, so the cardiologist has to set up the trolley, the haemodynamic monitoring equipment and contrast supply. Figure 5.1 shows the setup we use in Stoke in both labs.

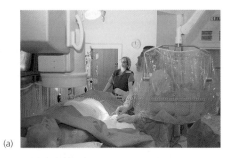

(a)

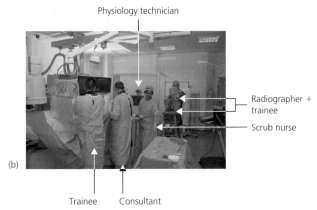

(b)

Figure 5.1 Catheter lab setup in Stoke.

In Figure 5.1a, the physiology technician is outside the room. This has advantages in terms of radiation protection but delays help in emergency situations. In Figure 5.1b, the physiology technician is in the room, but behind a lead protective screen.

It is important for the novice angiographer to ensure they are familiar with local practice. We recommend that before learning how to undertake angiography, they spend a session or two with the scrub nurses, learning how to set up and what is expected of an assistant. When on call, the staffing levels are reduced, and the operator may well be at the table alone.

Arterial and venous access techniques have been covered in Chapters 3 and 4.

Preparation of the access site

The area around the access site needs to be clear of hair, and this may necessitate shaving the area. You only need to shave an area sufficient to allow the adhesive area of the drape to stick without depilating the patient when the drape is removed.

The area should be washed, employing a no touch technique with chlorhexidine or a povidone iodine solution. In unstable cases, where the access site is the groin, it may be prudent to prepare both legs down to the knee in case an intra-aortic balloon pump is needed. Wipe off the excess antiseptic where the drape will stick, otherwise the back of the drape will not adhere to the skin and maintain the sterility of the working area.

Open the drape and place appropriately. Some packs have to be opened in the right way as the foot end is longer than the head end. Normally they have an arrow marked on the underside to guide correct placement.

Draw up and label your local anaesthetic and nitrate to reduce the risk of maladministration. Prepare some heparinized saline by diluting 1000 iu heparin in 500 mL of saline and use this for flushing equipment.

Take the manifold and connect the syringe to it. Connect the pressure tubing the port nearest the patient, the contrast tubing to the port nearest the syringe. Pass the other ends of both sets of tubing to a non-sterile assistant, who will connect to the pressure transducer and contrast reservoir. Draw the contrast through until the syringe is half full. Invert it so that the air is near the exit, and then expel all air in the syringe and manifold. The assistant should then flush the pressure tubing. This should leave an airless system; failure to do will leave air bubbles that may be injected with potentially fatal consequences. Figure 5.2a shows markedly reduced flow down a left anterior descending (LAD) in a non-dominant left coronary artery (LCA). Figure 5.2b shows actual bubbles inadvertently being injected in an intermediate artery.

> **Critical safety point**: Get into the habit of checking for air bubbles in the manifold.

The next step is to balance the pressure, to allow accurate assessment of intracardiac pressures. This should be performed at the level of the mid right atrium, which corresponds approximately to the level of the mid chest in an anteroposterior direction.

Take the catheter from the unscrubbed assistant, and flush it through with saline. Pass a J-tipped 0.038″ guidewire through the diagnostic catheter, until the tip of the wire approaches the end of the catheter. Pass the catheter and wire together, through the haemostatic valve on the arterial sheath. Fix the catheter and advance the wire until only 5 cm remains at the hub of the catheter, then advance it as one unit, holding both wire and catheter in the right hand and feeding through the sheath

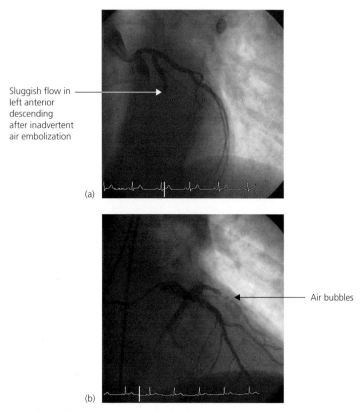

Sluggish flow in left anterior descending after inadvertent air embolization

(a)

Air bubbles

(b)

Figure 5.2 Air in the coronary circulation.

with the left. Start radiographic screening after only 40 cm has been introduced, or the wire does not pass easily. Advance the wire and catheter until the wire approaches the aortic root, then fix the wire and slide the catheter to above the sinotubular junction. Withdraw the wire, rolling it into three or four large loops. Allow blood to flow back from the hub of the catheter, and then connect up to the manifold by asking for the manifold to be flushed as you connect. Ensuring that you connect a fluid to fluid interface minimizes the risk of inadvertent air introduction. Finally, aspirate back into the syringe through the catheter to confirm no air is present in the closed system.

The key setting up stages are summarized in Table 5.1.

Table 5.1   Key setting-up stages

1. Shave
2. Antiseptic
3. Drape
4. Draw up nitrate, lignocaine (lidocaine)
5. Connect manifold
6. Balance pressure
7. Flush catheter
8. Introduce catheter

Acquisition skills

Once the catheter is engaged (see Chapters 3 and 4), the angiographer needs to acquire the image. The use of hand injections is almost universal for coronary artery and graft injections, but power injectors are used when the volume of contrast is too large, or the pressure required to inject is high, as in ventriculography and aortography. The use of power injectors is detailed in the section on left ventriculography and aortography later in this chapter.

Hand injection skills

The skill in this technique comes in injecting enough contrast to gain the information required versus overinjecting and causing complications. When you pick up the manifold, it is important to hold it with the syringe upward at 30° +, which allows any air bubbles to remain at the top of the syringe, and not to be injected into the patient (Figure 5.3).

The injection needs to fill the artery, causing some flashback of contrast into the aorta. The injection needs to have three phases; it seems obvious to say that it has a beginning, a middle and an end.

- The beginning of the injection needs to be smooth and to increase quite quickly. If it is too sudden, then the recoil will push the catheter out.
- The middle phase needs to be smooth, and this is where the vessel needs to fill with contrast with sufficient force to cause some reflux back into the aortic root, providing information about the ostium of the vessel.
- The end phase allows contrast to run out after injection has ceased, while still acquiring the image. This will demonstrate any staining or dissection where contrast holds up (Figure 5.4).

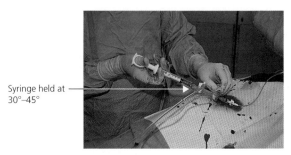

Syringe held at 30°–45°

Figure 5.3 Correct injection angle of 45°.

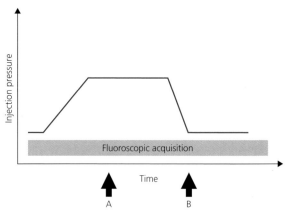

Figure 5.4 Pressure and time graph for appropriate injection. At point A contrast is seen to flush back past the catheter, indicating sufficient pressure. At point B vessel is fully filled, followed by acquisition to demonstrate vessel clearing.

Angiographic views – nomenclature

It is important to agree on common language to describe views that are taken to avoid confusion. The X-ray source is usually below the table and the image intensifier above the table. By convention, the terminology refers to the position of the image intensifier (II), not the X-ray source. Table 5.2 defines the standard terminology used for the orientation of

Table 5.2   Standard terminology for image intensifier orientation

Posterior anterior (PA)	The image intensifier is above the patient
Right anterior oblique (RAO)	The image intensifier is to the right of the patient, but above the level of the table
Left anterior oblique (LAO)	The image intensifier is to the left of the patient and above the level of the table
Cranial	The image intensifier is positioned towards the head end of the table
Caudal	The image intensifier is positioned towards the foot end
Left lateral	The image intensifier is at the level of the table, but on the left, and therefore the X-ray source is on the right
Right lateral	The image intensifier is at the level of the table, but on the right

the image intensifier, with the patient lying on the angiographic table and the operator standing to the patient's right.

Obviously if the image intensifier is positioned below the table, strictly speaking it should be termed a posterior oblique view, but most cardiologists will ask for an 'R/LAO' angulation, with a greater than 90° angle (i.e. left anterior oblique (LAO) 100°) for just beyond left lateral view. This is used in radial cases for achieving a modified left lateral view, since a conventional lateral cannot be obtained with the arm at the patient's side during a radial case.

Views can be a combination or right/left and cranial/caudal. By convention, the right/left is put first (i.e. RAO 30° cranial 30° would represent an angulation of 30° to the right from the vertical and 30° towards the head from the vertical.

Left ventriculography

The left ventricle (LV) is ideally placed for angiographic assessment, being easily accessed from the aortic root in most cases. Left ventriculography allows assessment of LV wall motion, ejection fraction, LV volumes and mitral valve regurgitation. There are few cases where it should not be performed, although crossing a severely diseased aortic valve to perform a left ventricular angiogram is not mandatory in the

Table 5.3   Absolute and relative contraindications to left ventriculography

Severe aortic stenosis	The risks of crossing a valve (i.e. embolization, perforation, thrombus on equipment) with a prolonged attempt at passage, etc. need to be weighed against the additional information that can be obtained. The additional risk may or may not be worth-while, but certainly will need consideration
Left-sided endocarditis	The risk of embolization makes this an absolute contraindication
Left ventricular clot	The risk of embolization makes this a relative contraindication. Unfortunately the operator is often not aware of the clot until the picture has been acquired. Large anterior infarcts with low flow states are particularly at risk and it is reasonable to avoid left ventricular angiography in these patients
Uncontrolled heart failure	May be made aggravated by contrast injection

era of reliable non-invasive imaging. Indications for left ventriculography include:

- Presence of coronary artery disease
- Assessment of mitral valve regurgitation
- Assessment of heart failure
- Assessment of ventricular septal defect.

There are firmly held opinions about whether the left ventriculogram should be performed prior to or after coronary angiography. The mere fact that cardiologists debate this point seems to indicate that neither is right or wrong. Now that most information that can be garnered at ventriculography can also be easily gained by non-invasive echocardiography, the need for ventriculography is lessening, and in certain circumstances – as detailed in Table 5.3 – ventriculography may be excluded.

Catheter selection

Whether access has been from the radial or femoral artery, the technique for crossing the valve is similar. The catheter selected is usually a pigtail (Figure 5.5), which has side and end holes to allow an adequate volume of contrast to exit the catheter, without the velocity of the jets being too great, which would increase the risk of ventricular perforation. Some pigtails are angled, which may provoke less ventricular ectopy.

Side holes

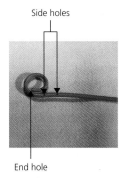

End hole

Figure 5.5 Pigtail catheter in close-up.

In aortic stenosis or hypertrophic obstructive cardiomyopathy, where the degree of left ventricular hypertrophy may be substantial, a pigtail catheter may provoke significant ventricular ectopy; in this situation a Gensini catheter can be used. This still has an end hole but fewer side holes and is relatively straight. However, in most cases of aortic stenosis, we would exchange the catheter used to cross the valve for a pigtail over a double length 0.035″ exchange wire.

Injector settings

Most power injectors allow individualization of three components of the injection: volume of contrast, maximum flow rate of contrast and the acceleration phase as the injection builds up to maximum flow rates. Typically the volume chosen will be between 30 and 45 mL. The flow rate will be between 10 and 15 mL/s and the acceleration phase or rate rise will be between 0.5 and 1 second.

The aim is to deliver the minimum amount of contrast required to gain diagnostic data. Injection of too small a volume of contrast or too slowly will underestimate valvular regurgitation and make assessment of LV function more difficult. Injection of too large a volume of contrast, at too high a flow rate or too rapid a rate rise will cause ventricular ectopy, increase the risk of VT or perforation, or cause catheter displacement back into the aorta. Some cardiologists use test shots of 5–10 mL of contrast.

Crossing the valve

There are a number of techniques available to the operator, one of which is to advance the pigtail catheter up to the valve in the right anterior oblique (RAO) 30° view. The catheter is rotated to be orientated towards 4–5 o'clock, as viewed by the operator on the viewing monitor. The J-shaped end of the wire is then advanced against the valve. If it does not slip straight across, continue to push until 3–4 cm of wire has curled back up in the sinus, then withdraw the catheter slowly until it is above the valve by 3 or 4 cm, and you are left with a gentle curve of wire. As you then withdraw the wire, it should prolapse across. If it does not, rotate the catheter by a quarter of a turn and try again. Sometimes getting the patient to take a deep breath in can help.

With a stenotic valve, the pigtail should again be the first catheter of choice. We would still use the J-shaped end of the wire, as this minimizes the chance of perforation of the valve. However a low threshold should be employed for changing to a straight wire. The technique with straight wire is to position the catheter 5–10 cm above the valve, directing the catheter towards 4–6 o'clock in the RAO 30° view. Then advance the wire towards the valve, aiming for the mid point of the aortic valve. With practice, it is possible to perceive when the tip of the wire is being buffeted by the high velocity aortic jet; aim for this point. If not successful, withdraw wire and catheter off the valve, rotate catheter by a small amount and advance again.

If the pigtail catheter is unsuccessful, alternatives include an AL2 (Amplatz left 2), as this has a good chance of success. Others use JR4 or multipurpose (MPA1) catheters with some success. Once across, as with any catheter that does not have side holes, a catheter exchange with a double length wire to a pigtail catheter may be useful to reduce risk of ventricular perforation.

Catheter exchange

This is really a two-person procedure early on in the training process. The catheter that has successfully crossed the valve is disconnected following pressure confirmation of being in the LV cavity. A double length wire is flushed in its housing and the J-shaped end is passed down the catheter until it appears in the LV cavity. The wire is fixed in position and the catheter is withdrawn back off the wire whilst screening to ensure that the wire tip remains in the LV cavity. This is crucial if any significant period of time has been spent getting it in position in the first place. Two operators are useful because it is difficult to screen, withdraw the catheter and feed the wire at the same time. It is worth practising this technique, perhaps when it has not been a struggle to get into the LV cavity, as it is not good practice to try something for the first time when losing catheter position would be disadvantageous. This may be the case if you attempt a catheter exchange when it has taken a significant period of time to cross the valve the first place.

The next step is to wipe the wire with a clean swab wet with saline and flush the pigtail catheter with heparinized saline. This is then advanced onto the wire and the procedure reversed. The wire is fixed, and screened to ensure it does not move, and then the catheter advanced into the LV cavity. Once in, the wire is withdrawn, then the pigtail catheter should be aspirated and flushed and connected to the power injector.

It should be remembered that it only takes a minute or two for thrombus to form on a guidewire in a non-anticoagulated patient. Every 2–3 minutes, the wire needs to be withdrawn and wiped, the catheter aspirated and flushed, to avoid thrombus formation (Figure 5.6a). This may manifest only as a damped pressure tracing (Figure 5.6b).

Catheter position in the left ventricular cavity

Once the catheter is in the LV cavity there are two important steps: the first is to get an adequate LV pressure trace to demonstrate LV end-diastolic pressure (LV EDP); the second is to position the catheter correctly to maximize the information from the LV angiogram. Positioned too distally, it will underestimate the degree of mitral regurgitation and provoke ventricular ectopics. Positioned too proximally, it will over-estimate or provoke spurious mitral regurgitation. The apex may also be suboptimally opacified, which may in turn reduce diagnostic accuracy regarding apical thrombus and wall motion abnormalities.

The ideal position is one in which the pigtail portion of the catheter is placed at the level of the papillary muscles, which is usually mid-cavity level (Figure 5.7). If the pigtail catheter is seen to dip or twist with each beat, then it may be entangled in the subvalvar apparatus and requires repositioning.

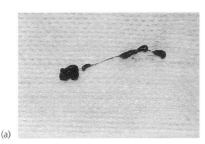

(a)

Figure 5.6   (a) Thrombus from catheter equipment.

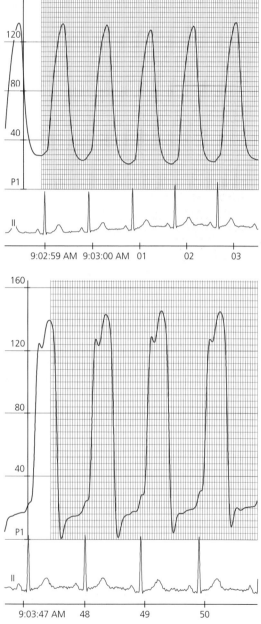

Figure 5.6 (*Continued*) (b) Damped (top) and normal (bottom) left ventricular pressure trace.

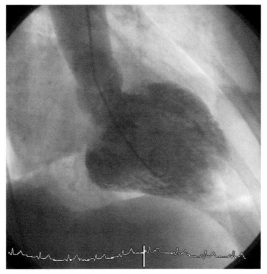

Figure 5.7   Pigtail position in the left ventricular cavity.

Once the haemodynamic information is obtained, the pressure line is disconnected, and the high-pressure connector from the power injector is taken. The large syringe is primed to form a meniscus of contrast at the end and connected to the pigtail catheter. The powered injector is then reversed so that blood is drawn back into the syringe, removing any trapped air from the line. The power injector is then set and armed.

Angiographic views

Two views are used:

1. A straight RAO between 30° and 40°, the exact angle depending on the manufacturer of the angiographic software, as it will have been calibrated for a particular RAO angulation to allow calculation of LV volumes and therefore ejection fraction.
2. Typically LAO 50–60°; some would argue that a small amount of cranial angulation allows better assessment of the septum. Biplane labs make this easy, without increasing the burden of contrast. However, in most centres with monoplane labs, many cardiologists accept a single RAO view as an assessment of LV function.

Once set up, the operator should initially warn the patient that they may experience a hot flush, which is related to contrast-induced vasodilatation. The patient may also get a sensation of passing urine via the same mechanism. Many patients find this acutely embarrassing and it can cause great anxiety if they are not warned about it.

The operator should ask the patient to breathe in, as this pulls the diaphragm out of the way, allowing time for the radiographer to position the table and acquire the picture. An assistant normally operates the power injector, although some centres have an operator-controlled foot pedal. The acquisition run should continue until the ventricle is clear of contrast.

The high-pressure tubing should then be disconnected and the pressure manifold reconnected. The pigtail catheter can then be withdrawn to the aortic root, with continuous pressure measurement. This gives a pullback gradient across the aortic valve, providing three measurements: (1) the peak-to-peak drop from LV to aorta, (2) the mean pressure difference between LV and aorta, which is electronically derived from the integral of the area under the left ventricular minus aortic pressure curves, and (3) the calculated aortic valve area (see Chapter 9: catheterization formula).

Complications of left ventriculography

Complications of left ventriculography include:

- Arrhythmia such as ectopics, ventricular tachycardia and ventricular fibrillation
- Myocardial staining – contrast being injected intramyocardially, which is most often seen with an end-hole catheter
- Myocardial perforation
- Contrast complications
- Embolization of air or thrombus.

Left ventricular wall motion and ejection fraction

WALL MOTION

The RAO and LAO projections of the left ventricle are divided into five segments each (Figure 5.8a,b). The RAO 30° is divided into the anterior basal and anterior apical, the apex, the inferobasal and inferoapical segments (Figure 5.8a, panels 1 and 2). The LAO 50–60° view is divided into the basal septum, apicoseptum, apex, apicolateral and basolateral segments (Figure 5.8a, panels 3 and 4). All can move normally, be hypokinetic (move less than normal) or akinetic (not move at all) or dyskinetic (move the wrong way). A segment may move normally but be delayed, and this is termed dyssynchronous. The cardiologist should assess regional wall motion as well as gross overall function – graded normal, mild, moderate and severely impaired.

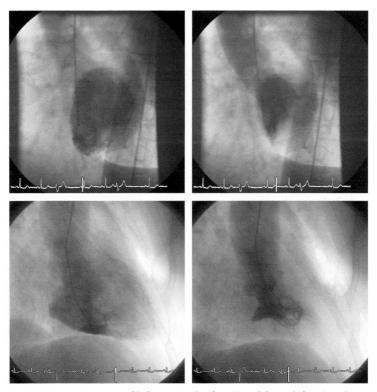

Figure 5.8 Assessment of left ventricular function. (a) Top left: Diastole (left anterior oblique), top right: systole (left anterior oblique), bottom left: diastole (right anterior oblique), bottom right: systole (right anterior oblique).

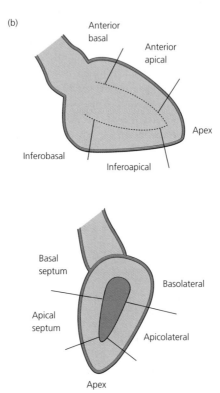

Figure 5.8 (*Continued*) (b) Right anterior oblique (top) and left anterior oblique (bottom).

LEFT VENTRICULAR VOLUME

This is usually generated by software incorporated in the angiographic viewing system. It involves using an internal calibration constant, usually two dots on the screen compared with an external known dimension, conventionally the internal diameter of the catheter.

This technique is subject to a number of limitations. The most obvious is the skill in interpreting where the border of the LV ends, as the automatic edge detection software is not always reliable and tends to overestimate LV volumes. If LV volumes are to be assessed, even at a later date offline, do not move the table during the acquisition of the left ventriculogram. LV end-diastolic volume (EDV) is

Table 5.4 Factors that may over- and underestimate mitral regurgitation

Overestimate	Coexisting aortic stenosis
	Pigtail too close to mitral valve
	Pigtail caught in mitral subvalvar apparatus
	Ectopic activity
Underestimate	Inadequate ventriculogram (not enough contrast or too slowly injected)
	Grossly dilated left ventricle
	Pigtail placed too distally

definitely abnormal when $>110 \, mL/m^2$ and LV end-systolic volume (ESV) $>45 \, mL/m^2$.

EJECTION FRACTION

This is dependent on the calculation of the maximum LV volume (LV EDV) and the minimum LV volume (LV ESV). This allows the calculation of the ejection fraction:

$$EF = (LV \, EDV - LV \, ESV)/LV \, EDV$$

However most cardiologists will use a simple visual assessment of overall LV function.

Assessment of mitral regurgitation

The left ventriculogram can be used to grade the severity of mitral regurgitation. However, there are a number of limitations, and certain factors will over- or underestimate mitral regurgitation (Table 5.4).

Mitral regurgitation can be graded in two ways, either on a four-point scale or as mild, moderate and severe. It is usually assessed on the third beat/cardiac cycle after contrast enters the LV cavity. The presence of ectopics makes assessment more difficult, but most would assess the third beat after an ectopic as well (Figure 5.9):

- *Mild*: The jet is thin, but may be highly penetrating. The contrast that enters the left atrium is cleared with each beat.
- *Moderate*: The atrium is filled, and contrast builds up with successive beats. However it is never as dense as the LV.

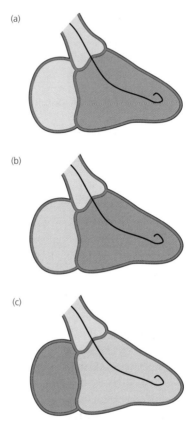

Figure 5.9 Assessment of mitral regurgitation. (a) Mild: Fails to opacify left atrium. (b) Moderate: Fully fills left atrium but density is less than left ventricle. (c) Severe: Fully fills left atrium but density is greater than left ventricle.

- *Severe*: The atrium fills completely and pulmonary veins may be seen. The density of contrast in the left atrium is greater than that of the LV.

Aortography

The aorta is easily assessed by cardiac catheterization techniques. However, cross-sectional imaging with computerized tomography (CT) and cardiac magnetic resonance (CMR) have better resolution and have

Table 5.5   Indications and contraindications for aortography

Indications	Presence of significant, long standing hypertension
	Increased likelihood of aortic root dilatation
	Assessment of aortic valve regurgitation
	Assessment of patients needing larger than expected catheters for coronary angiography
	Aortic syndromes
	Marfan's syndrome
	Coarctation
	Aortic dissection: CT and MRI are better and safer
	Supravalvular aortic stenosis – CT and MRI have better resolution
Contraindications: absolute and relative	Aortic valvular endocarditis. The risk of embolization makes this a contraindication
	Uncontrolled heart failure, which may be made worse by the contrast injection

replaced angiography in the assessment of aortic root calibre, the degree of calcification, and the location of aortic root plaque disease.

Echocardiography is also supplanting aortography in the assessment of aortic valve function, giving excellent estimates of the degree of aortic stenosis and regurgitation. Currently the only real role for aortography is to provide information regarding the degree of aortic regurgitation and gross aortic root size in two dimensions.

The indications and contrainidications for aortography are listed in Table 5.5.

Catheter selection and placement

Whether access has been from the radial or femoral route, the catheter usually selected is a pigtail, given the advantages of high flow rates associated with a larger number of exit holes and lower jet velocities. However, recoil backwards is often significant with a pigtail and may lead to an underestimation of aortic regurgitation (AR). Some operators recommend a Gensini catheter, which has four side holes and an end hole. We advise placing the tip of the chosen catheter at the level of the sinotubular junction, or just above the coronary arteries, as placing it too proximally will underestimate the degree of AR.

Injector settings

Typically, the volume injected will vary between 40 and 60 mL. The flow rate will be between 15 and 25 mL/s and the acceleration phase or rate rise will be between 0.5 and 1 second. The aim is to deliver the minimum amount of contrast to gain useful diagnostic data. Underinjecting will underestimate valvular regurgitation.

Angiographic views

There are two main projections: LAO 50–60° and RAO 30–40°. In a biplane lab it is worth acquiring both, but in a monoplane lab most cardiologists will settle for the LAO view alone, although either is acceptable. The exception to this is when it is necessary to assess the aortic arch where the RAO view sees this in profile, but is opened right out in the LAO 50–60° view.

Assessment of aortic regurgitation

There are a number of factors that can lead to inaccurate assessment of aortic regurgitation. These are listed in Table 5.6.

Aortic regurgitation is usually graded either on a four-point numerical scale or as mild, moderate and severe. It is usually assessed on the third beat after contrast. Ectopics are rare and better quality pictures are usually obtained (Figure 5.10a,b):

- *Mild*: The jet is thin, but may be highly penetrating. The contrast enters the left ventricle, but is cleared with each beat.

Table 5.6 Factors that may over- and underestimate aortic regurgitation

Overestimate	Pigtail too close to aortic valve
Underestimate	Inadequate contrast study
	Not enough contrast
	Too slow an injection rate
	Inadequate rate rise
	Grossly dilated aortic root
	Pigtail placed too proximally

- *Moderate*: The ventricle is filled, and contrast builds up with successive beats, but it is never as dense as the aorta.
- *Severe*: The ventricle fills completely within one beat, and the density of contrast in the left ventricle is greater than that of the aorta.

(a)

(i)

(ii)

(iii)

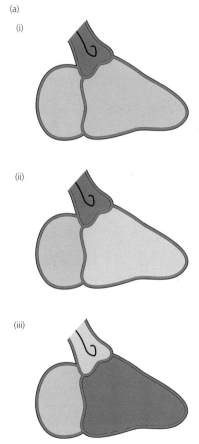

Figure 5.10 Assessment of aortic regurgitation. (a) (i) Mild: Penetrating jet at aortic regurgitation which fails to fill left ventricular cavity. (ii) Moderate: Aortic regurgitation fills cavity but density is less than aorta. (iii) Severe: Aortic regurgitation fills cavity but density of left ventricle exceeds aorta.

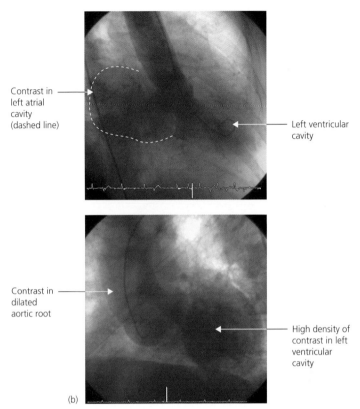

Contrast in left atrial cavity (dashed line)

Left ventricular cavity

Contrast in dilated aortic root

High density of contrast in left ventricular cavity

(b)

Figure 5.10 (*Continued*) (b) Moderate/severe mitral regurgitation and severe aortic regurgitation.

Coronary angiography

Nomenclature

- Ostial: The point of origin of the vessel
- Proximal: The first section of the vessel
- Distal: The last section
- Bifurcation: Point where branch arises from parent vessel
- Side branch: The vessel that arises from a main artery. For example in an LAD bifurcation, the side branch would be the resulting diagonal.

Table 5.7   Indications for varying catheter selection

Initial catheter likely to be too small	Very tall patient
	Long standing hypertension
	Significant aortic regurgitation
Initial catheter too large	Very small patient
	Upward left main stem take-off

In the figures relating to standard angiographic views for LCA and RCA, each view is taken from the same patient, labelled (patient A). Additional panels are included to demonstrate the difference in dominant and non-dominant arteries.

Left main stem

The main stem is a critically important vessel. It may be the first vessel intubated during the routine cardiac catheterization procedure and subtends a large myocardial territory. The presence of severe ostial left main stem (LMS) disease will have major implications for the rest of the study.

CATHETER SELECTION

Radial catheter selection is discussed in Chapter 3. Femoral catheter selection is covered in more depth in Chapter 4, but the basics are outlined here.

The initial catheter would be a Judkins (JL4). If this is too small, usually indicated by the catheter sitting above the LMS in the left coronary sinus in the LAO view or to the left and above in the LAO caudal view, then the catheter should be upsized by one size to a JL5 or JL4 for a radial procedure.

If the catheter is too big, sitting below and to the right the main stem in the sinus, then it should be downsized by one size. Most labs will carry JL3.5, 4, 5 and 6 (Table 5.7).

Amplatz catheters are useful if the origin of the main stem is pointing more downwards, or the root/sinus is very dilated. Most labs will carry Amplatz 1–3.

TECHNIQUE

See radial (Chapter 3) and femoral (Chapter 4) access chapters.

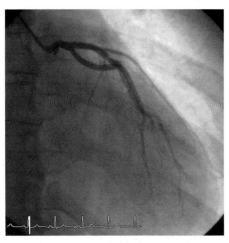

Figure 5.11   Posteroanterior view of the left coronary artery (Patient A).

VIEWS

In the event that the test shot reveals a normal ostium and a non-critical distal left main lesion then a full run of views can be taken.

- *Posteroanterior (PA)*: This gives a good view of the LMS including the ostium, and some operators regard it as the first view. Sometimes shallow RAO or LAO is needed to remove the density of the spine from the picture, as this may overlap with the LMS (Figure 5.11). PA caudal is an alternative.
- *LAO 40–50° cranial 20–25°*: This view gives good information about the ostium and the mid LMS, but often foreshortens the bifurcation. Sometimes increasing the degree of cranial angulation allows better imaging of the distal LMS and bifurcation. Figure 5.12 demonstrates the difference between dominant and non-dominant circumflex (Cx) arteries. In Figure 5.12a the posterior descending (PD) artery lines up with the LAD, whereas in Figure 5.12b it terminates well before this point.
- *LAO 40° caudal 20–40°*: This gives a good view of the entire length of the left main and usually of the bifurcation (Figure 5.13, page 162).
- *Straight RAO 20–40° views*: These will give information regarding the mid portion of the main stem (Figure 5.14, page 163).

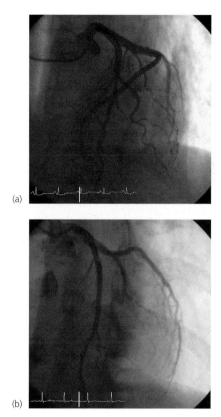

Figure 5.12 Left coronary artery (left anterior oblique cranial view).
(a) LCA dominant; (b) LCA non-dominant (Patient A).

Critical left main stem coronary artery disease

The first clue to the presence of this may be pressure damping on engagement, which is why the pressure trace should be inspected as the catheter is first engaged. In the event that the initial test shot demonstrates very severe ostial LMS disease, then it is prudent to limit the number of acquisition runs that are performed. The trauma of intubation with the catheter and the proaggregatory effects of contrast can provoke an LMS occlusion. Unfortunately this complication may be delayed, occurring 20–30 minutes post procedure.

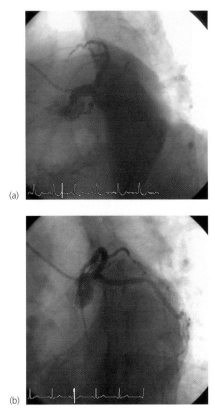

Figure 5.13 Left coronary artery (left anterior oblique view). (b) Patient A.

However it is still essential that enough diagnostic information is obtained to allow an appropriate management plan to be developed. First this means proving beyond reasonable doubt that the LMS disease is real, and not artefactual and due to a suboptimal injection. Second, it is necessary to demonstrate what target arteries there are for surgical or percutaneous revascularization.

It is prudent to limit the acquisition runs to LAO cranial, RAO caudal and LAO caudal. These three views will give you key information regarding main stem, LM bifurcation and LAD/Cx status. Occasionally, only the first two may be achievable, because of haemodynamic instability or ECG changes.

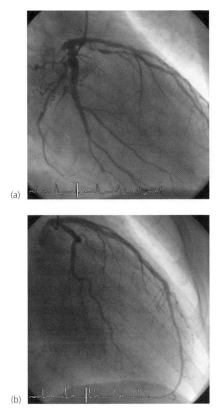

(a)

(b)

Figure 5.14 Left coronary artery (right anterior oblique view). (b) Patient A.

CRITICAL LMS DISEASE VIEWS

Two views are essential in LMS disease and one is considered optional:

- LAO 50 cranial 25° (essential)
- RAO 30 caudal 10° (essential)
- LAO 40 caudal 30° (optional)

Pressure damping describes the phenomenon where catheter tip pressure falls on intubation of the artery or becomes ventricularized. A ventricularized pressure trace looks similar to the trace one would expect from the LV, and represents partial occlusion of the vessel (Figure 5.15).

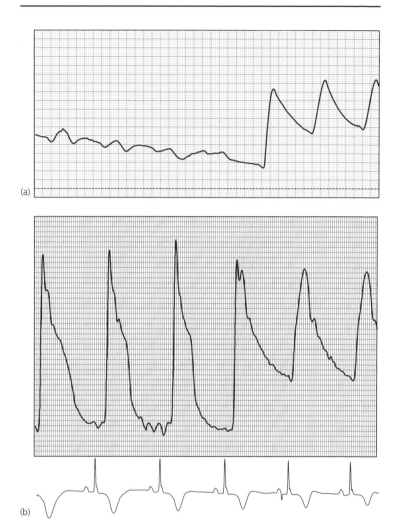

Figure 5.15   (a) Damped and (b) ventricularized pressure traces.

The catheter should be gently disengaged and then be reintroduced and placed below the LMS. It may be worth increasing the French size of the catheter to ensure that the main stem cannot be intubated and occluded by the catheter, or alternatively reducing the French size of the catheter so that the main stem can be engaged without occluding it. A series of non-selectively engaged views may be taken. An alternative is to increase the size of the curve of the catheter (i.e. from a JL4 to a JL5 etc.) to allow the tip to be placed slightly away from the ostium.

Table 5.8   Indicators suggesting critical ostial left main stem disease

Preprocedural indicators	Marked peripheral vascular disease
	Global ischaemia on stress testing or rest angina
	Hypotension on stress testing
	Syncope on effort
On-table indicators	Pressure damping
	Ventricularization of the catheter tip pressure

Unless faced with haemodynamic collapse, there is no reason not to take enough views to make a diagnostic decision and one view is usually insufficient.

The indicators suggestive of critical ostial LMS disease are listed in Table 5.8. In the presence of critical ostial LMS disease it is prudent to approach the RCA with caution. Similarly it may be sensible to assess the LV non-invasively by transthoracic echocardiography to further limit the risk of procedure-induced complications.

Left anterior descending artery

LEFT MAIN BIFURCATION/PROXIMAL LEFT ANTERIOR DESCENDING ARTERY

The LM bifurcation is best seen either in a very steep LAO cranial (i.e. LAO 40–50° with 35°+ cranial or an LAO 40° caudal 40° view).

PROXIMAL LEFT ANTERIOR DESCENDING

The proximal LAD runs from the bifurcation of the LMS to the origin of the first septal artery. It is well seen in a number of views, although some views will better demonstrate the anatomy in some patients than in others.

Typical views may include LAO 40–50° cranial 25° and a standard RAO 40° caudal 20–30° view. Sometimes an LAO caudal or PA caudal 20–30° will show the very proximal segment. On occasion, with an intermediate vessel overlapping the LAD, an LAO 70° cranial 30° or RAO 60° caudal 10–40° helps.

MID LEFT ANTERIOR DESCENDING

The mid LAD is usually well seen in most LAO cranial views – both LAO 10° cranial 40° and the more traditional LAO 50° cranial 25°. It is also seen in most RAO cranial views (i.e. RAO 40° cranial 30° (Figure 5.16).

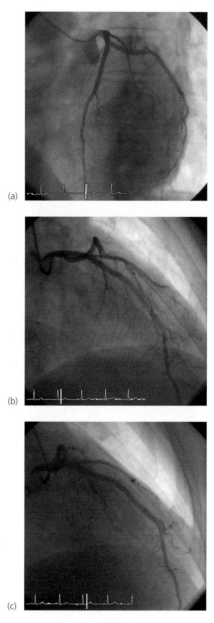

Figure 5.16 (a) Anteroposterior cranial, (b) shallow right anterior oblique cranial (RAO 10° cranial 30°) and (c) steep right anterior oblique cranial (RAO 30° cranial 30°) views of the left anterior descending artery (Patient A).

The lateral is also very useful (Figure 5.17). The cranial views are useful in distinguishing diagonal disease, especially the LAO 50° cranial 25° where the septal arteries will go to the left of the viewing monitor and the diagonals will go to the right as viewed by the operator.

DISTAL LEFT ANTERIOR DESCENDING

We use the lateral and RAO 40° cranial 30° views for the distal LAD. The LAO 50° cranial 25° view is also useful. Standard and alternative views are summarized in Table 5.9.

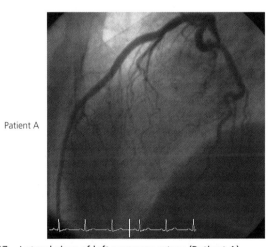

Patient A

Figure 5.17   Lateral view of left coronary artery (Patient A).

Table 5.9   Summary of left anterior descending (LAD) views

Vessel segment	Standard view	Alternative views
Left main bifurcation	LAO cranial, LAO caudal	
Proximal LAD	LAO cranial, RAO caudal	LAO caudal, PA caudal, steep LAO cranial, steep RAO caudal
Mid LAD	LAO cranial, RAO cranial, lateral	
Distal LAD	RAO cranial, lateral	LAO cranial

LAO, left anterior oblique; RAO, right anterior oblique; PA, posteroanterior.

Circumflex artery

LEFT MAIN BIFURCATION AND PROXIMAL SEGMENT

The LM bifurcation views are exactly the same as the LAD bifurcation discussed in the previous section.

PROXIMAL CIRCUMFLEX

The proximal Cx is foreshortened in most of the cranial views, although the ostium may be seen in profile in the LAO 50° cranial 25° view sometimes. The traditional views for this part of the Cx would be LAO 50–60° or an LAO caudal. As the image intensifier comes round to the PA and RAO caudal views, the proximal Cx begins to foreshorten again. However, these views are well worth reviewing in the presence of circumflex disease.

Intermediate artery origins are usually well seen in the straight LAO or LAO 40° caudal 20–40° view, or occasionally the PA caudal 25° (Figure 5.18).

MID CIRCUMFLEX

The mid Cx and origin of the obtuse marginal vessels are well seen in PA caudal 20–30° and RAO 40° and RAO 30–40° caudal 20–30° (Figure 5.19, page 170). These views also usually show the body of the intermediates and early obtuse marginal (OM) vessels.

DISTAL CIRCUMFLEX

The distal atrioventricular (AV) groove Cx is sometimes clearly seen in the LAO cranial view, especially if the artery is dominant. This view can really open out the Cx/PD artery junction. We use a standard LAO 50° cranial 25° view. Sometimes an RAO cranial can achieve the same end in a dominant left-sided circulation. Some typical Cx views are summarized in Table 5.10.

Right coronary artery

The RCA may be a vestigial vessel of no consequence or may be very large, supplying most of the inferior and lateral wall. Some indication about the relative size will be gained from the area covered by the LCA.

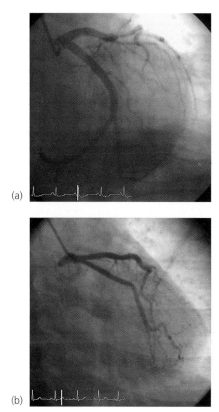

(a)

(b)

Figure 5.18 Anteroposterior view of left coronary artery. (a) Dominant left coronary artery. (b) Non-dominant left coronary artery, Patient A.

CATHETER SELECTION

Most RCAs can be intubated with a Judkins JR4 catheter. The technique is described in the radial and femoral access chapters. However, if that fails it can be much more difficult to select an alternative that will selectively engage the RCA ostium. The most common reason for not engaging with a JR4 is an aberrant anterior location. In this situation, a Williams catheter or a modified right Amplatz will offer some success. If these are unsuccessful, a left Amplatz 0.75, 1 or 2 may be tried.

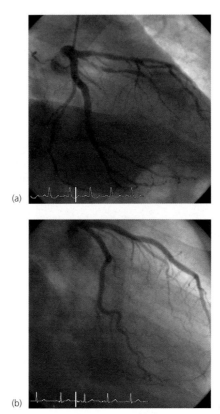

(a)

(b)

Figure 5.19 Right anterior oblique view of left coronary artery. (a) Co-dominant circumflex. (b) Patient A.

Table 5.10 Summary of typical circumflex views

Vessel segment	Standard view	Alternative views
Left main bifurcation	LAO cranial, LAO caudal	
Proximal Cx/intermediate origin	LAO, LAO caudal	LAO cranial RAO caudal
Mid left anterior descending/OM origin/ OM body	LAO caudal, PA caudal, RAO and RAO caudal	
Distal Cx/posterior descending	LAO cranial	RAO cranial

LAO, left anterior oblique; RAO, right anterior oblique; PA, posteroanterior; OM, obtuse marginal; Cx, circumflex.

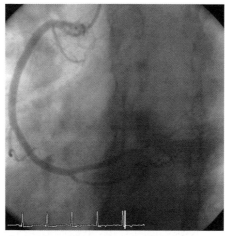

Figure 5.20 Left anterior oblique view of right coronary artery (Patient A).

OSTIUM AND PROXIMAL RIGHT CORONARY ARTERY

The RAO view foreshortens the RCA, and is essentially useless for the proximal vessel. The ostium is well seen with LAO 40° caudal 20° (Figure 5.20), and also usually well seen with a straight LAO 30–50° (Figure 5.21). Sometimes a lateral is quite helpful.

MID RIGHT CORONARY ARTERY

The mid RCA is well seen with a straight LAO, straight RAO (Figure 5.22) and a lateral (Figure 5.23, page 173).

DISTAL RIGHT CORONARY ARTERY

The distal RCA is seen well with an LAO 30° cranial 20° or straight PA cranial 20–30° (Figure 5.24, page 174). A lateral view will also often clearly demonstrate the distal vessel.

POSTERIOR DESCENDING AND POSTEROLATERAL BRANCHES

These branches are seen with the same view as the distal RCA, although sometimes an RAO cranial may show the posterolateral branches well. Typical RCA views are summarized in Table 5.11, page 174.

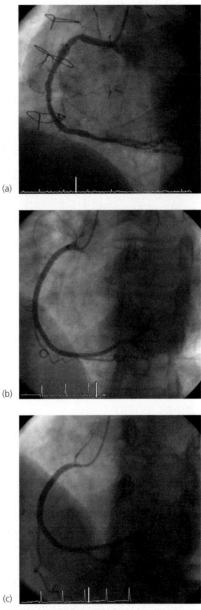

Figure 5.21 Left anterior oblique view of right coronary artery. (a) Left anterior oblique. (b) Left anterior oblique (Patient A). (c) Left anterior oblique cranial (Patient A).

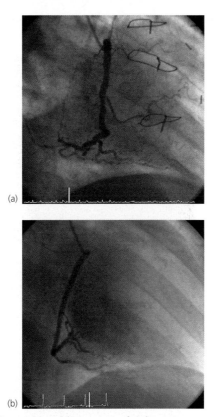

(a)

(b)

Figure 5.22 Right anterior oblique view of right coronary artery. (a) Right anterior oblique. (b) Right anterior oblique (Patient A).

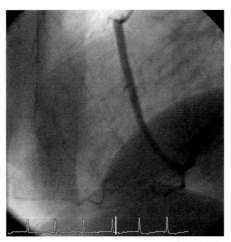

Figure 5.23 Lateral view of right coronary artery (Patient A).

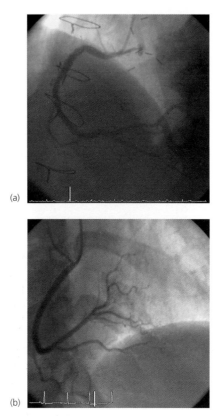

(a)

(b)

Figure 5.24 Posteroanterior cranial view of right coronary artery.
(a) Posteroanterior cranial view. (b) Posteroanterior cranial view
(Patient A).

Table 5.11 Summary of typical right coronary artery views

Vessel segment	Standard view	Alternative views
Right coronary artery ostium	LAO, LAO caudal	
Proximal right coronary artery	LAO, lateral	PA cranial
Mid right coronary artery	LAO, RAO and lateral	PA cranial
Distal right coronary artery/ posterior descending	LAO cranial, PA cranial	RAO cranial, lateral

LAO, left anterior oblique; RAO, right anterior oblique; PA, posteroanterior.

Atrial septal defect

Angiographic assessment of atrial septal defects (ASDs) is no longer the norm, and echocardiography and CMR give superior anatomical information, even in the current age of device closure. Most ASDs are single and relatively central, reflecting that two-thirds are secundum defects, a quarter are probably primum defects and the remainder are sinus venosus defects. This means that the default treatment is likely to be device closure. The role of the catheter lab in the assessment of ASDs is the calculation of the size of the shunt (see Chapter 6 for right heart catheterization technique and Chapter 9 for shunt calculations). However, occasionally an ASD may inadvertently be crossed during right heart catheterization, in which case it is worthy of further assessment, as it may be nothing more than a probe patent foramen ovale (PFO).

ATRIAL SEPTAL DEFECT STRATEGY

The first step is to confirm that the catheter is in the left atrium by obtaining a saturation, which should be >95 per cent. Exchange for a Gensini catheter and perform either a firm hand or motorized injection of a low volume (15–20 mL) and 10 mL/s to opacify the ASD. This needs to be done in LAO 40–50° with cranial 20–30° tilt, which places the septum in profile, rather than *en face*.

On withdrawal, a good-quality pressure trace is needed from left atrial to right atrial, to show pressure equalization between the two atrial chambers. A pulmonary angiogram may then be performed (volume 30–40 mL, flow rate 10–15 mL/s) (see Chapter 6). It is important to continue the acquisition run, because the purpose of the shot is not for pulmonary artery anatomy, but to confirm normal pulmonary venous drainage. This is performed in the PA projection.

Obviously a full saturation run is critical, to allow the site step-up to be accurately determined, and the size of the shunt calculated.

Ventricular septal defect

Ventricular septal defects (VSDs) are normally picked up earlier than ASDs because of the presence of a murmur. However, a number, including post-myocardial infarction (MI) VSDs are picked up later. In the acute MI setting, few interventions will have an impact on the very poor outcome seen in these patients. However in the stable situation of a congenital VSD or late survivor post MI with a VSD, angiography has a role.

VSD STRATEGY

The main caveat here is that left ventriculography is usually contraindicated in patients with a post-infarct VSD, who are or have been haemodynamically unstable in the recent past.

In non-infarct VSDs the left ventriculogram is the key. It needs to be acquired in the LAO 40–50° with cranial 20–30° tilt. This puts the septum in profile and will allow assessment as to where in the septum the shunt is occurring. The power injector should be set at a volume of 35–40 mL with flow rate of 12–15 mL/s. An RAO ventriculogram should also be obtained for assessment of function, and to confirm the flow of contrast in the pulmonary artery which lies anteriorly to the aorta (Figure 5.25). Figure 5.25a shows the flow of contrast into the pulmonary artery from an LV angiogram. Figure 5.25b is an LAO view of the same VSD and shows the track of contrast across the septum, normally seen in cross-section in this view.

A full saturation run is important to assess where in the RV there is the greatest step up and to allow a shunt severity calculation to be performed.

Patent ductus arteriosus

Patent ductus arteriosus is usually located just distal to the origin of the left subclavian artery. The vast majority of cases are picked up in childhood, but some are still recognized in adulthood. Closure can be achieved by either percutaneously delivered coils in a small ductus, percutaneously delivered device closure in a larger one or surgically by video-assisted thoroscopy.

The diagnosis is made by identifying a step up in the saturation in the pulmonary artery (usually the left pulmonary artery). However, because there is usually inadequate mixing, the shunt calculation is prone to error. It may be overestimated if the sample is taken within the jet derived from the aorta.

PATENT DUCTUS ARTERIOSUS STRATEGY

Angiographic assessment is usually a combination of right and left heart catheterization. The right heart normally involves trying to pass a

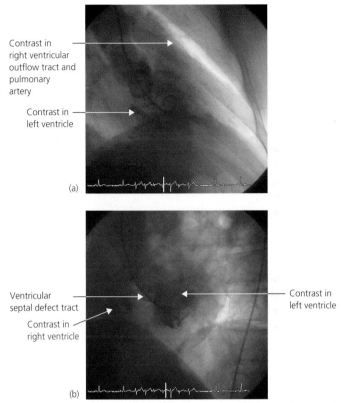

Contrast in right ventricular outflow tract and pulmonary artery

Contrast in left ventricle

(a)

Ventricular septal defect tract

Contrast in right ventricle

Contrast in left ventricle

(b)

Figure 5.25   Angiographic image of ventricular septal defect from a left ventricular angiogram. (a) Right anterior oblique view; (b) left anterior oblique view.

catheter across the defect, after a full saturation run. Logically, as the ductus is a continuation of the pulmonary artery and aorta, a reasonably straight catheter, such as a multipurpose A2, should pass easily. Then exchange for a Gensini or pigtail, and acquire the angiographic information with the catheter *in situ*.

The acquisition should be in the lateral view, as this allows sight of the ductus as it comes forward from the aorta to the main pulmonary artery/left pulmonary artery junction. The power injector settings should be set at a volume of 35–40 mL with a flow rate of 20 mL/s, as the aim is anatomical identification.

Interpretation

Classifying coronary artery disease severity

ANGIOGRAPHIC CRITERIA – VISUAL CLASSIFICATION

Anatomical description can be used to stratify the likelihood of procedural success at percutaneous intervention (PCI). A visual classification was adopted by the American Heart Association and American College of Cardiology in 1988 [1] (Table 5.12). This was developed in the pre-GPIIb-IIIa inhibitor and stent era, but remains a valid classification. The easy transportation of DICOM CD images has made descriptive classifications less important for the decision-making process regarding PCI, but it remains useful for the classification of procedural risks.

Nevertheless, there are certain limitations to a visual reporting system, including that it relies on observer interpretation and therefore there is likely to be a degree of interobserver variability. There are problems with agreeing on accessibility, length, eccentricity and the degree of angulation. Type B characteristics are all equally weighted, but only the degree of calcification, occlusion and the presence of thrombus have been consistently associated with an adverse outcome.

ANGIOGRAPHIC ASSESSMENT OF CORONARY FLOW

There are three common methods of assessing coronary flow: (1) epicardial (macrovascular) coronary flow assessed by thrombolysis in myocardial infarction (TIMI) flow rates, (2) epicardial coronary flow assessed by TIMI frame counts and (3) microvascular blood flow assessed by TIMI myocardial perfusion grade (myocardial blush).

TIMI flow rates

This is a very useful, easily applied classification of epicardial (macrovascular) coronary flow and was developed from the TIMI 1 trial [2] (Figure 5.27, page 181; Table 5.13, page 182). Its original application was as a mechanism for classifying the response to thrombolysis, but it is equally well applied to pre/post-PCI procedures and the effect on coronary flow of severe coronary artery stenoses. The severity of a coronary stenosis is not the only determinant of TIMI flow, which can also be slow because of poor run-off owing to of distal embolization, slow following balloon inflation and also because of microvascular

Table 5.12 American Heart Association and American College of Cardiology classification of coronary lesion morphology

Type	Characteristics	Success rate
Type A (Figure 5.26a)	Discrete <10 mm Concentric Readily accessible Angulation <45° Little calcification No thrombus No significant side branches Smooth contour	High rate of primary success (> 85%) and are low risk procedures (~2%)
Type B (Figure 5.26b) B1 = 1 type B characteristic; B2 = 2 or more type B characteristics	Tubular (10–20 mm) Eccentric Moderate tortuosity pre-lesion Angulation between 45 and 90° Irregular lesion >Moderate calcification Occlusion <3 months old Ostial lesion Bifurcation with two wires Thrombus	Moderate success (60–85%) and are moderate risk procedures (~10%)
Type C (Figure 5.26c)	Diffuse (>20 mm) Very tortuous run-in Angulation >90° Occlusion >3 months Unprotected side branches Vein grafts	Low success (<60%) and high risk (~21%)

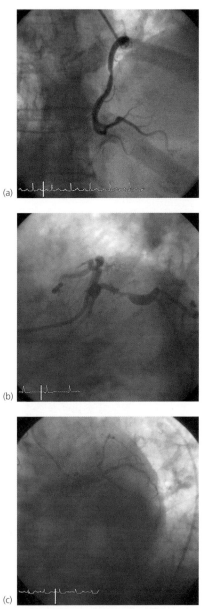

Figure 5.26   (a) Benestent type A lesion. (b) This is a type B lesion in circumflex because the angulation is between 45 and 90° and there is calcification. (c) Bifurcating distal left main shows type C lesion because of unprotected side branches type C lesion.

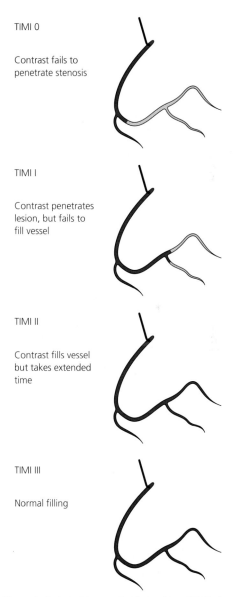

TIMI 0

Contrast fails to
penetrate stenosis

TIMI I

Contrast penetrates
lesion, but fails to
fill vessel

TIMI II

Contrast fills vessel
but takes extended
time

TIMI III

Normal filling

Figure 5.27   Thrombolysis in Myocardial Infarction (TIMI) flow grades.

Table 5.13 Thrombolysis in myocardial infarction (TIMI) flow grades

TIMI flow	Characteristic
0	No contrast seen to flow through the stenosis
I	Contrast penetrates the stenosis, but does not fill the vascular tree
II	Contrast fills the vascular tree beyond the stenosis, but is slower than prestenotic segments and clears more slowly
III	Normal flow with prompt filling and emptying of the vascular tree

Adapted from [2].

coronary disease. Similarly, non-culprit arteries are used to provide the standard of flow against which to judge culprit arteries. It has been shown that flow in non-culprit arteries is reduced post MI.

There is often disagreement about the classification of TIMI II flow. This is important as it is associated with adverse events following MI.

TIMI frame count

TIMI flow grading has been criticized for being subjective and categorical, but this is also its strength (i.e. its ease of application). In an attempt to reduce variability, TIMI frame counting was developed [3], although it is not used widely except in research settings. The aim was to standardize the number of frames of cine film required for contrast to reach standardized distal coronary landmarks. The first frame used is when a column of contrast extends across the full width of the artery, the contrast touches both borders at the origin of the artery and there is antegrade flow. The last frame used is when contrast first passes the distal landmark, when full opacification distally is not needed. The landmarks used are as follows:

- *LAD*: The most distal branch of the LAD or if the LAD wraps around the apex, the branch closest to the apex. The LAD value is divided by 1.7 to correct for its increased length when compared to the RCA and Cx.
- *Cx*: The artery chosen is the one with the longest total distance which still passes through the lesion. If two arteries have similar length, the more distal of the two is used. The actual endpoint is the terminal branch of that artery.
- *RCA*: The first small branch after the origin of the PD artery in the crux artery is the RCA endpoint. If the lesion is in the PD artery, the first branch after the lesion is used instead.

Table 5.14 Thrombolysis in Myocardial Infarction (TIMI) myocardial perfusion grade

Grade	Characteristics
TMP 0	Minimal or no blush
TMP 1	Blush appears , but is slow to clear. Contrast staining is present at 30 seconds
TMP 2	Blush is delayed both in entry and exit. Contrast strongly persists beyond the 'washout period' of three beats
TMP 3	Normal entry and exit of contrast with normal blush. Contrast has either gone entirely or is minimally present after the washout phase

Adapted from [4].

The normal value lies between 15 and 27 frames at 30 frames per second acquisition rate. Obviously, if the acquisition frame rate is different, then the normal values will also change.

TIMI myocardial perfusion grade

Improved epicardial blood flow demonstrated by improved TIMI flow grades or frame count are associated with reduced mortality after myocardial infarction treated with thrombolysis. Microvascular perfusion can also be assessed angiographically by the appearance of a ground-glass appearance during contrast injection, often called myocardial blush. This has been standardized as the TIMI myocardial perfusion grade (Table 5.14) [4]. TMP 3 has been shown to be a better predictor of outcome than TIMI III flow grade and can substratify TIMI III flow into high and low risk groups according to the presence or absence of TMP 3 (Figure 5.28).

Glossary of angiographic terms

See Table 5.15.

Bifurcation lesions

Bifurcation lesions, along with chronic total occlusions, remain the Achilles heel of the interventional cardiologist. This is driven mainly by the additional complexity of the intervention, which increases the

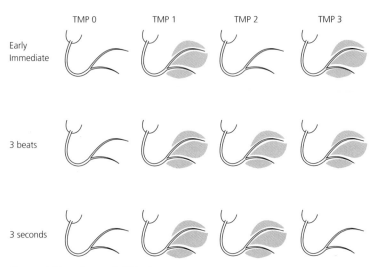

Figure 5.28 Myocardial blush.

procedural risk, and the increased incidence of restenosis, the maladaptive healing process that leads to recurrence of ischaemic symptoms due to intimal proliferation.

Bifurcation lesions are classified as prebranch, postbranch, parent vessel, true bifurcation and ostial (Figure 5.31), but this is only important in the strategy for any planned coronary intervention. A more recent classification is simpler and more intuitive and marks a stenosis as present or absent in the form of a binary code: 1 means disease is present and 0 means it is not. Then using a three-number system, the parent vessel, continuation vessel and side branch are classified. For example 1,1,1 would mean that parent vessel, continuation vessel and side branch all have disease. 1,0,1 would tell us that the parent and side branches are affected. However, it is important to view the lesion from the point of view of both treatment strategies – surgery and PCI. Current feelings in intervention suggest that simpler strategies are the way forward, even in the era of drug eluting stents (DES), and many complex stenting techniques are again falling out of favour. Nevertheless, the emergence of newer, specifically designed stents, with drug coatings to reduce the unacceptable levels of restenosis that remain with traditional stent designs, even with DES, will act again as an impetus to try to get on top of bifurcation lesions.

Table 5.15 Glossary of angiographic terms

Feature	Definition
Eccentricity	A stenosis that lies in the outer quarter of the vessel, or where the lesion is apparent in one view, but markedly underestimated in orthogonal views
Irregularity	
Ulceration	A crater in the lesion that does not extend beyond the outer wall of the vessel
Intimal flap	An extension of the vessel wall into the lumen; associated with a double lumen or an abrupt loss of calibre (see separate subclassification of dissection lesions)
Aneurysmal dilatation	A segment of artery wider than the reference calibre of the vessel
Sawtooth pattern	Multiple lesion
Lesion length	Measured using a view that minimizes foreshortening
Discrete	<10 mm
Tubular	10–20 mm
Diffuse	>20 mm
Ostial	Within 3 mm of the ostium
Lesion angulation	The angle between the prelesion length and postlesion length
Moderate	45–90°
Severe	>90°
Bifurcation stenosis	A >1.5 mm vessel originates from within the stenosis (see separate subclassification of bifurcation lesions)
Lesion accessibility	
Moderate tortuosity	Lesion is distal to two >75° bends
Severe tortuosity	Lesion is distal to three >75° bends
Degenerated vein graft	Graft is diseased for more than 50% of its length
Calcification	
Moderate	Calcified vessel only seen on movement
Severe	Calcium visible on a static image (Figure 5.29)
Total occlusion	TIMI 0 or I flow
Thrombus	Discrete intraluminal filling defect, which can be seen as distinct from vessel wall. Staining may be present but is not necessary (Figure 5.30)

Adapted from [5].

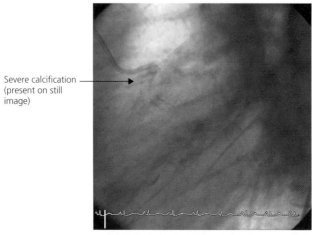

Severe calcification (present on still image)

Figure 5.29   Severe coronary calcification.

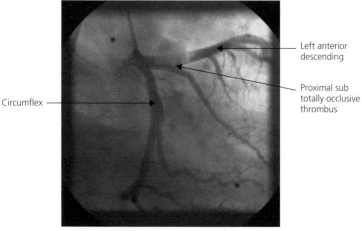

Left anterior descending

Proximal sub totally occlusive thrombus

Circumflex

Figure 5.30   Thrombus in left anterior descending artery.

There are one or two commonly accepted rules:

- Side branches less than 2 mm are often not treated by PCI, nor are they grafted at coronary artery bypass graft (CABG) operations. They may occlude at PCI if the susbsequent point applies, but if they do, it may be associated with a small troponin rise and is usually well tolerated.

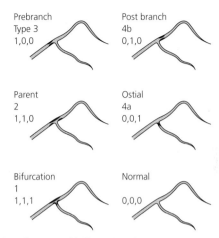

Prebranch
Type 3
1,0,0

Post branch
4b
0,1,0

Parent
2
1,1,0

Ostial
4a
0,0,1

Bifurcation
1
1,1,1

Normal
0,0,0

Figure 5.31 Classification of bifurcation disease. 1,1,1 system: parent, continuation, side branch. 1 – disease present; 0 – disease absent.

• Side branches with lesions of 50 per cent or less rarely occlude, especially if they are larger than 2 mm in calibre. The exception to this occurs where the parent vessel lesion is very bulky and atheromatous material can be pushed into the side branch (a process described as snowploughing) causing it to occlude, even if it was angiographically normal.

Coronary dissection

Coronary dissections have a number of aetiologies and can be iatrogenic, such as those caused by catheter tips or angioplasty wires (Figure 5.32), or spontaneous [6]. However, the most common dissection is probably the dissection that is related to a primary plaque event. The clinical course of all dissections is difficult to predict, and their haemodynamic stability cannot be relied upon. This is especially true for catheter tip dissections, which are usually ostial and are directed antegradely and therefore in line with the direction of coronary flow, which can cause further propagation of the dissection plane. Increasingly dissections are being stented, even if they are not haemodynamically significant, because this scaffolds the dissected segment back against the vessel wall and allows it to heal and re-endothelialize. Dissections that

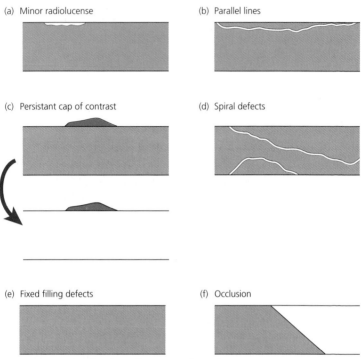

(a) Minor radiolucense

(b) Parallel lines

(c) Persistant cap of contrast

(d) Spiral defects

(e) Fixed filling defects

(f) Occlusion

Figure 5.32 Classification of coronary dissections.

are >50 per cent of the lumen calibre or that restrict flow are regarded as severe and warrant treatment. These are classified A–F (Figure 5.32):

- A – Minor lucencies within the lumen, with persistent contrast
- B – Parallel lines within the lumen, but with no contrast holding up at the end of the run
- C – Persistent extraluminal cap with contrast holding up outside the normal lumen
- D – Spiral defects
- E – Fixed filling defect, which persist
- F – New total occlusions.

Thrombus

The angiographic appearance of thrombus can be quite varied and Figure 5.30, page 186, shows a number of different appearances of thrombus in the coronary artery. Typically, in the context of an acute coronary syndrome the vessel is occluded and may look as if it has abruptly terminated, without any tapering segment. However thrombus may also appear as a haze with suboptimal blood flow or as a relatively fixed filling defect.

References

1. Ellis SG, Vandormael MG, Cowley MJ *et al.* Coronary morphologic and clinical determinants of procedural outcome with angioplasty for multivessel coronary disease. Implications for patient selection. Multivessel Angioplasty Prognosis Study Group. *Circulation* 1990; **82:** 1193–1202.
2. Sheehan FH, Braunwald E, Canner P *et al.* The effect of intravenous thrombolytic therapy on left ventricular function: a report on tissue-type plasminogen activator and streptokinase from the Thrombolysis in Myocardial Infarction (TIMI Phase I) trial. *Circulation* 1987; **75:** 817–829.
3. Gibson CM, Cannon CP, Daley WL *et al.* TIMI frame count: a quantitative method of assessing coronary artery flow. *Circulation* 1996; **93:** 879–888.
4. Gibson CM, Cannon CP, Murphy SA *et al.* Relationship of TIMI myocardial perfusion grade to mortality after administration of thrombolytic drugs. *Circulation* 2000; **101:** 125–130.
5. Lansky A and Popma J. Qualitative and quantitative angiography. In: Topol EJ, ed. *Textbook of Interventional Cardiology*, 3rd edn. Philadelphia: WB Saunders, 1999, pp. 725–747.
6. Butler R, Webster MW, Davies G *et al.* Spontaneous dissection of native coronary arteries. *Heart (British Cardiac Society)* 2005; **91:** 223–224.

Non-coronary angiography 6

Right heart catheterization

Access to the right heart has been described in Chapters 3 and 4, which outline the venous access techniques from the superior route using the antecubital fossa and inferior access via the femoral vein. Other superior venous access sites such as internal jugular and subclavian punctures are covered in other texts and are usually well-established skills in the cardiac trainee. There are situations where one route may be preferable to the other (Table 6.1).

The indications, contraindications and complications of right heart catheterization are summarized in Table 6.2.

Techniques

There are two major techniques available, each of which has their proponents: balloon flotation catheters and end hole catheters.

FLOTATION CATHETER

This technique is uses the principles of the catheter designed by Drs Swan and Ganz. It consists of a catheter with two lumens, one originating distally at the tip of the catheter and the other more proximally,

Table 6.1   Clinical situations suggesting an access route preference

Access route	Better for
Femoral vein	Right femoral artery puncture
	Easier simultaneous access
	Routine right heart catheter
	Poor upper arm venous access
	Intravenous cannula phlebitis, multiple venepunctures, etc.
	Superior vena cava thrombosis
	Temporary pacing wires
	Thoracic outlet syndrome
Superior (brachial, subclavian, internal jugular)	Femoral or iliac vein thrombus
	Anticoagulation
	Caval filter
	Pulmonary hypertension
	Gross right heart enlargement

Table 6.2   Indications, contraindications and complications of right heart catheterization

Indication	Assessment of mitral valve disease
	Assessment of pulmonary hypertension
	Unexplained dyspnoea
	Assessment of right-sided valvular disease
	Shunt assessment in congenital heart disease
	Pericardial disease
Contraindication	Pulmonary oedema and unable to lie flat
	Pulmonary haemorrhage
	Right heart thrombus/vegetation/tumour
Complication	Pulmonary artery dissection/rupture
	Right ventricular/right atrial rupture
	Arrhythmia: atrial fibrillation, right bundle branch block, ventricular extrasystole, atrioventricular block or ventricular tachycardia
	Tricuspid or pulmonary valve damage

the location of which should theoretically at least, place it in the right atrium in most adults. There is a distal thermistor that allows cardiac output assessment to be made and a balloon inflation port (Figure 6.1).

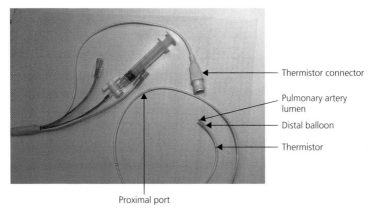

Thermistor connector

Pulmonary artery
lumen

Distal balloon

Thermistor

Proximal port

Figure 6.1 Balloon-tipped catheter in close-up.

Each lumen is flushed with heparinized saline and then capped off. The balloon is tested *ex vivo* by inflating it with a prespecified amount of air. The manifold/pressure line is balanced at the level of the mid chest, which should be equivalent to the level of the mid right atrium. The catheter is then introduced. Once the distal tip is seen in the right atrium (RA), the balloon is inflated. A loop is made in the RA, with the catheter tip gradually being advanced across the valve orifice, until it is caught by the tricuspid inflow and carried across. Once across, clockwise torque is applied to allow the tip to point upwards towards the pulmonary outflow tract. Sometimes a little traction helps with twisting motion. It is then advanced, the balloon (hopefully) carrying the catheter across the pulmonary valve and into the pulmonary artery.

Occasionally, the balloon will not cross one or other valve, in which case use an 0.025″ guidewire to stiffen the catheter and pass it that way. If using a larger calibre catheter than the traditional Swan–Ganz catheter, then the use of a standard 0.035″ wire is possible. Often the key is the clockwise torque once across the tricuspid valve, combined with a degree of simultaneous traction, which takes the large curve off the catheter but does not pull it back across the tricuspid valve. As the catheter straightens, it will often advance upwards towards the right ventricular outflow tract.

A balloon-tipped catheter should not be advanced into a wedge position with the balloon deflated, as the catheter may inadvertently advance into a vessel that is too small to accommodate the inflated balloon and cause potentially fatal pulmonary haemorrhage from the resulting barotrauma.

The flotation catheter can be advanced with its balloon inflated into a distal pulmonary artery to measure the pulmonary capillary wedge pressure, and thereby give an indirect measurement of left atrial pressure. This should be confirmed by withdrawing blood from the wedged position and demonstrating an O_2 saturation of >95 per cent along with a typical pressure trace. In practice it can be difficult to withdraw blood back through the lumen of the flotation catheter when it is wedged. It is worth using gentle negative pressure on the syringe, and allowing the blood to come back slowly, otherwise you can collapse the capillary bed and get nothing back. Any of the four main lobes can be used, although balloon catheters tend to enter right lower.

The balloon is then deflated, and a sample drawn into the catheter for O_2 saturation and withdrawn to the main pulmonary artery (MPA), for pressure recording and saturation sampling and directed to the other pulmonary artery for sampling there. The catheter can then be withdrawn for pressure recordings and saturation sampling.

END HOLE CATHETER

The advantage of this technique is that the catheters are stiffer and more easily torqued. The major disadvantage is that obtaining an accurate wedge pressure is significantly harder. The most commonly chosen catheter is the multipurpose (MPA1 or Cournand), but others are available. Side holes make it more difficult to obtain a wedge trace if they are located too distal from the tip (i.e. an NIH or MPA2 catheter).

Prior to touching the catheter you need to balance the manifold or pressure line. In right heart catheterization, where small pressure errors may prove important, extra care needs to be taken. If simultaneous pressures are needed, for instance in mitral stenosis or answering a question regarding constriction/restriction, it is very important that both arterial and venous pressure lines are balanced together at exactly the same height.

The catheter is prepared in the standard way (i.e. flushed, connected to a pressure line or manifold and flushed again). It is then introduced from the venous sheath, without a guidewire. We employ screening for catheter advancement, as it will tend to enter branches of the inferior vena cava on the way up to the heart. When the catheter enters the RA, there are a number of options for trying to enter the right ventricle (RV).

If coming from the groin, MPA1 catheters sometimes pass straight across the tricuspid valve, in a manner similar to temporary pacing wires. Otherwise you need to pass it through the valve. There are two major techniques: the first is to direct the tip of the catheter towards 9–11 o'clock on the screen, until it touches the lateral wall of the RA. Then advance the catheter so that it begins to form a loop in the RA. When the loop is formed, gradually withdraw the catheter, so that the tip is gradually withdrawn. It should then prolapse across the tricuspid valve. The alternative technique is to initially place the catheter towards 1–3 o'clock, and then repeat the process by forming a loop. Occasionally introducing a 0.038″ guidewire changes the dynamics, and it can cross the tricuspid valve on its own followed by the catheter. Once in the RV, the catheter is twisted clockwise to direct it to the RV outflow tract. Sometimes, a little traction is needed, as well as clockwise torque, to make the catheter turn into the RV outflow tract and then advance upwards. The catheter should then pass through the RV outflow tract, through the pulmonary valve and into the MPA. The wedge is achieved by asking the patient to take a deep breath in and advancing the catheter into a peripheral vessel. The wedge is obtained when the waveform changes from PA trace to typical wedge.

Pressure waves

The pressure waves in the right heart can help with identification of the location of the catheter tip, as the catheter position on the screen may be confusing. The waveforms are critical for some diagnostic decision making.

During the normal right heart study, we often proceed directly to obtain the wedge pressure (PCWP), and perform the saturation run and pressure trace recordings on the way back out, although some operators will perform saturations on the way in.

To achieve simultaneous pressure recordings for the transmitral pressure gradient, a pigtail catheter is placed in the left ventricle. It is important to reiterate that if simultaneous pressures are anticipated, ensure both pressure lines are balanced together to minimize the risk of error in any resulting calculation.

RIGHT ATRIAL PRESSURE TRACE

In the normal subject RA contraction increases pressure, which is called an *a* wave (Figure 6.2). The *c* wave is a small deflection noted on

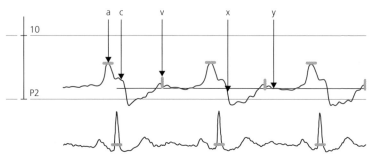

Figure 6.2   Right atrial pressure trace.

the *a* wave. This is thought to be either closure of the tricuspid valve or the onset of ventricular systole, which are almost simultaneous events. The initial descent after the *a* wave is called the *x* descent, which is mediated by RA relaxation and downward movement of the tricuspid valve. Following this is the *v* wave, which represents RA filling during ventricular systole. The *y* descent follows the *v* wave and represents rapid filling of the RV after opening of the tricuspid valve.

RIGHT VENTRICULAR PRESSURE TRACE

This is shown in Figure 6.3.

PULMONARY ARTERY PRESSURE TRACE

The dicrotic notch on the descent of the PA pressure trace (Figure 6.4) represents pulmonary valve closure.

WEDGE

The wedge represents a measurement of the indirect left atrial pressure trace. It will also have *a*, *c* and *v* waves and *x* and *y* descents. The limitations of the wedge pressure trace are described below. In Figure 6.5 an indirect pressure trace was obtained using standard technique with a non-balloon end hole catheter (Figure 6.5a, page 198). However there was also an atrial septal defect (ASD) present which allowed a direct measurement of left atrial (LA) pressure in the same patient (Figure 6.5b). In this example the wedge underestimates direct LA pressure.

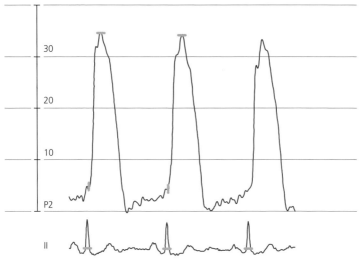

Figure 6.3   Right ventricular pressure trace.

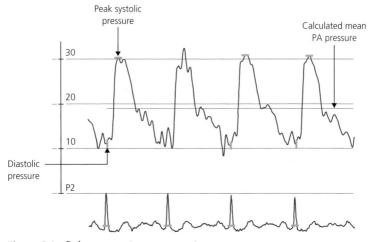

Figure 6.4   Pulmonary artery pressure trace.

Limitations of wedge pressure

The basic premise of the wedge pressure is that it approximates the LA pressure when measured directly through a trans-septal puncture. The

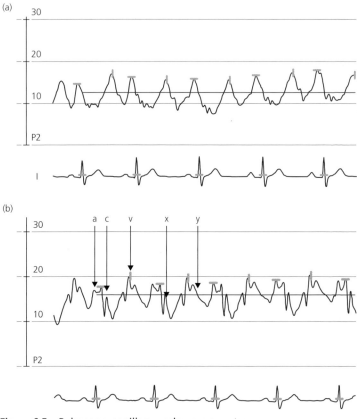

Figure 6.5   Pulmonary capillary wedge pressure trace.

wedge is always slightly out of phase with the left ventricle (LV) pressure and direct LA pressure, as it is measuring the pressure some distance from its generation. This is only important in simultaneous pressure measurement for mitral valve gradients.

As discussed, in Figure 6.5 the catheter crossed a small ASD, allowing a direct assessment of LA pressure (Figure 6.5a), which can be compared to the wedge pressure trace (Figure 6.5b) from the same patient. The *a*, *c* and *v* waves are marked, along with the *x* and *y* descents. In this example there is no respiratory variation because of the ASD. The *a* wave represents atrial contraction, the *c* wave represents the percussion wave from the onset of ventricular systole and the *v* wave represents

Table 6.3   Pulmonary capillary wedge pressure (PCWP): validity and technical limitations

Conditions where PCWP is less valid	Chronic obstructive pulmonary disease with pulmonary hypertension
	Pulmonary venoconstriction/pulmonary vein stenosis
	Left ventricular failure
	Severe mitral valve disease (balloon-tipped catheter)
Technical limitations	Inadequate wedge trace: Try to reposition the catheter. A small contrast injection should hold up demonstrating the pulmonary vessels beyond the injection site for 10–15 seconds, without being washed out
	Lumen too small: Use bigger catheter with larger lumen
	Line partially obstructed with thrombus: Change line/catheter – do not try to flush it through!

passive venous filling with the tricuspid valve shut. The x descent is due to atrial relaxation and the y descent represents tricuspid opening.

The validity and technical limitations of PCWP are listed in Table 6.3.

Pressure considerations

High v wave on PCWP can occur in mitral regurgitation, post CABG, in VSD and in any infiltrative process. It is not very specific for mitral regurgitation (MR). The presence of MR should be confirmed by ventriculography or echocardiography.

PRESSURE WAVEFORM EXAMPLES

Mitral stenosis

Pure mitral stenosis remains relatively uncommon in the UK, unless there is a significant local migrant population from an area where rheumatic fever has been endemic. Towards the latter stages of the disease process, patients who have had rheumatic fever are often dyspnoeic. They may have palpitations, which are related to atrial fibrillation in more than 50 per cent of cases. However this represents the end of a progressive, life-long disease which may have had a latent period of 20+ years from the time of the acute rheumatic episode to onset of symptoms. The 10-year survival is of the order of 50–60 per cent, with most deaths being due to heart failure or embolic events.

Mitral stenosis is the major valvular reason for which right heart catheterization is undertaken and a critical part of the procedure is to

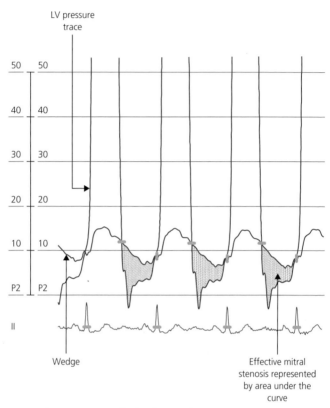

LV pressure trace

Wedge

Effective mitral stenosis represented by area under the curve

Figure 6.6   Pressure trace of mitral stenosis.

obtain a high-quality, stable PCWP trace, as this will make interpretation/calculation of gradients easier (Figure 6.6). Most patients with significant mitral stenosis are in atrial fibrillation, so the *a* wave will be absent and there will be significant beat-to-beat variation in the gradient. Therefore it is imperative to have simultaneous LV and wedge pressure. Transthoracic and transoesophogeal echo offer significant anatomical advantages, but the tests are complementary rather than mutually exclusive, as echocardiography does not give an assessment of pressure.

The mean mitral valve area is the shaded area on Figure 6.6, and represents the pressure differential between atrium and ventricle. If cardiac output is calculated, then this measurement can give the estimated mitral valve area (Table 6.4).

Table 6.4   Severity of mitral stenosis by mitral valve area and transmitral gradient

	Mitral valve area/cm^2	Mean transmitral gradient/mmHg
Normal	4–6	0
Mild	1.5–4	0–5
Moderate	1.0–1.5	5–10
Severe	<1.0	>10

Mitral regurgitation

Mitral regurgitation has a much more mixed aetiology and is related to:

• Ischaemic heart disease
• Ruptured chordae
• Annular dilatation
• Myxomatous degeneration
• Mitral valve prolapse.

The patients will tolerate slowly progressive MR for a long time, but acute severe MR, which may be seen in the context of myocardial infarction, will present very quickly with haemodynamic compromise. Chronic MR has a prolonged asymptomatic phase followed by more rapid decline with increasing dyspnoea which corresponds with progressive ventricular dilatation and pulmonary hypertension. Transthoracic and transoesophogeal echo represent the best imaging modality for assessing MR, as they can give an assessment of the reparability of the valve.

In Figure 6.7 the abnormal area is within systole and consists of a giant *V* wave. There is no accompanying mitral stenosis in this example and the PCWP and LV overlap during diastole. The MR is assessed better by left ventriculography and echocardiography than by any assessment of the pressure trace.

Aortic stenosis

Aortic stenosis is often a slowly developing chronic condition, where the gradient progressively increases by 5–12 mmHg per year, corresponding to a decline in the valve area of 0.1 mm^2 per year. The patient may have a long latent asymptomatic phase, during which the LV will hypertrophy in order to maintain cardiac output. Eventually the LV can no longer overcome the obstruction, and symptoms such as angina,

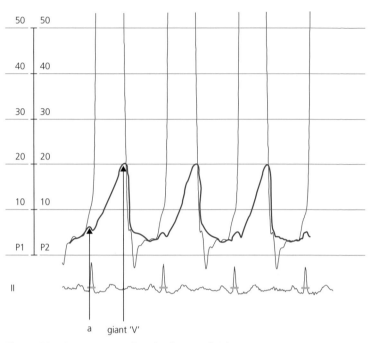

Figure 6.7   Pressure trace in mitral regurgitation

Table 6.5   Causes of aortic stenosis

Young to middle-aged adults	Calcification and fibrosis of congenitally bicuspid aortic valve
	Rheumatic aortic stenosis
Middle aged to elderly	Senile degenerative aortic stenosis
	Calcification of bicuspid valve
	Rheumatic aortic stenosis

heart failure and syncope will develop. The onset of symptoms is a poor prognostic sign. The causes of aortic stenosis vary with age (Table 6.5).

The mean aortic gradient is the hatched area in Figure 6.8. Realistically, cardiologists rarely attempted to obtain simultaneous LV and aortic pressure, as it would entail needing either a two-port catheter with proximal and distal measuring ports for simultaneous pressure or performing a septal puncture and passing the catheter from RA through LA to LV. The risk of septal puncture far outweighs the

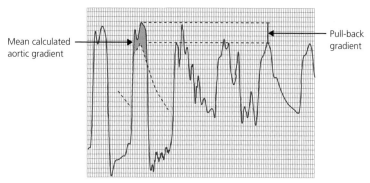

Figure 6.8 Pressure trace in aortic stenosis.

Table 6.6 Severity of aortic stenosis by aortic valve area and transaortic gradient

	Aortic valve area (cm²)	Peak to peak transaortic pull-back gradient (mmHg)
Normal	>1.4	0
Mild	1.2–1.4	<25
Moderate	1.0–1.2	25–60
Severe	0.8–1.0	60–100
Critical	<0.8	>100

disadvantages of manipulating the timing of the pressure recoding. Most cardiologists in the UK settle for a direct pull-back gradient.

The classification of aortic stenosis according to aortic valve area and transaortic gradient is shown in Table 6.6.

Aortic regurgitation

The causes of aortic regurgitation include:

- Bicuspid valve
- Rheumatic disease
- Infective endocarditis
- Trauma
- Aortic root dilatation (hypertension, Marfan's syndrome, aneurysm, dissection, syphilis).

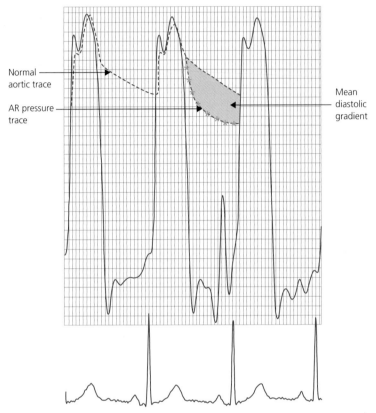

Normal aortic trace

AR pressure trace

Mean diastolic gradient

Figure 6.9   Aortic pressure trace.

Aortic regurgitation may also have a long latent phase, but once the ventricle can no longer cope with the volume and pressure overload, progressive ventricular dilatation and progressive breathlessness ensues. It is beloved of examiners because of the high-volume pulse pressure, which generates classical clinical features that have acquired eponymous names.

In reality, we very rarely perform a right heart catheter for aortic regurgitation. The plot of LV and aortic pressure traces is interesting (Figure 6.9), but rarely used for decision-making processes because echo gives more easily interpretable results.

Right heart assessment for pericardial constriction and myocardial restriction

Determining the major underlying cause of haemodynamic compromise in an unwell patient can be very difficult, and differentiating between restriction and constriction is particularly so. The role of echocardiography is also very important, but sometimes direct and simultaneous pressure measurement may help, either giving the diagnosis or added diagnostic certainty to the echocardiographic suspicion.

PERICARDIAL CONSTRICTION

Pericardial inflammatory disease can ultimately lead to scarring of both visceral and parietal pericardium, currently most commonly due to recurrent viral pericarditis. It is usually patchy. Historically a major cause was tuberculosis, where the heart could become encased in a thickly scarred, fibrotic pericardium. Other causes may include postcardiac surgery, systemic inflammatory diseases, neoplasms, chronic renal disease and radiation exposure (i.e. radiotherapy).

Pericardial constriction is characterized by systemic and pulmonary venous hypertension, and the concomitant symptoms and signs of pulmonary and peripheral oedema and a raised jugular venous pressure (JVP). Once pressure in the systemic and pulmonary veins reaches 20–30 mmHg, orthopnoea and paroxysmal nocturnal dyspnoea will begin to appear. The classical clinical sign is a paradoxical increase in the JVP on *inspiration* (it normally falls with a breath in).

An important role for cardiac catheterization still remains in these conditions, despite the progress in echocardiography, and both techniques are complementary in this situation.

Set-up should be meticulous, and the catheters should be balanced together to ensure that baselines are equal. The right and left ventricular end diastolic pressures are usually elevated and also within 5 mmHg of each other. The only caveat to that is that atrial contraction may alter the pressure trace in either chamber, so the assessment of pressure equivalence should either be pre *a* wave or at the very end of diastole.

Atrial pressures (RA and PCWP as an indirect measure of LA pressure) may differ if there is significant tricuspid regurgitation (TR) or MR. Pulmonary arterial pressure may be normal or mildly raised, but significant pulmonary hypertension usually indicates other coexisting pulmonary or valvular heart disease.

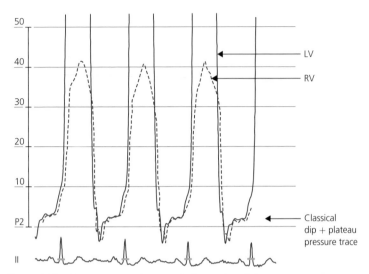

Figure 6.10 Pressure trace in constrictive pericarditis.

The simultaneous right and left ventricular pressure trace is typical (Figure 6.10). The hallmark of constrictive pericarditis is the matching of RV and LV pressure traces. There is often an overshoot in the downstroke of both RV and LV pressure traces at the end of systole, before the more classical plateau in mid and late diastole – the square root sign.

RESTRICTIVE PATTERN

This is undoubtedly difficult and there is a lot of crossover between the haemodynamic picture of pericardial constriction and myocardial restriction.

The major causes are amyloid, haemochromatosis, radiation and infiltration. A lot of imaging can be achieved by echo and cardiac magnetic resonance (CMR), and these investigations may provide enough information to make a diagnosis. CMR is especially useful in the differentiation of infiltrative processes.

Haemodynamic pattern

After normal setup, including careful attention to simultaneous balancing of right and left pressure manifolds, a pigtail should be placed in the LV and an end-hole catheter, such as an MPA1 (Cournand), placed

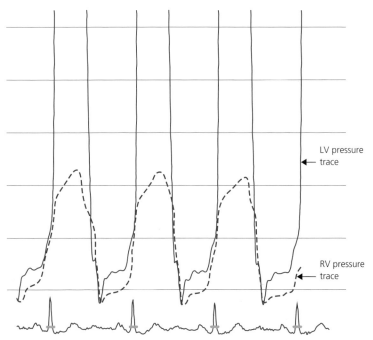

Figure 6.11 Left and right ventricular pressure traces in restrictive cardiomyopathy.

in the RV at mid cavity level. It is important to make sure that there is the minimum of ectopic activity to allow stable recordings, although sometimes a postectopic pause in a tachycardic subject may provide useful information in terms of the left and right ventricular end-diastolic pressures.

The LV pressure is normally slightly higher than the right, but they parallel each other very closely (Figure 6.11). Pulmonary arterial hypertension is more common, and presents at a more severe level ~40–50 mmHg.

Perhaps the most useful test is on deep inspiration (Figure 6.11). In predominantly myocardial restrictive disease, there are usually concordant changes in LV and RV pressure (i.e. both fall). However, with a predominantly constrictive pattern, there is a discordant pattern, with RV pressure increasing and LV pressure falling. Simplistically, this can be put down to the fixed volume of the pericardium and therefore both ventricles, so an increase in one ventricle has to lead to a decrease in the other. As this marked volume limitation does not exist in restrictive disease, this effect is not seen.

Pulmonary angiography

The usefulness of pulmonary angiography has gradually declined as the availability of high-quality cross-sectional imaging techniques such as computerized tomography (CT) and magnetic resonance imaging (MRI) has increased. CT can obtain good-quality images very rapidly, especially with multislice technology, although at the expense of an increase in X-ray dose. Similarly, with advances in gating technology, which allows MRI to acquire images more slowly but with less artefact by selecting the acquisition according to the ECG signal, good-quality images can be produced even in patients with atrial fibrillation (AF).

Cross-sectional imaging techniques remain the province of the radiologist in most UK centres, but occasionally the cardiologist is called upon to perform pulmonary angiography, usually in the context of acute, life-threatening pulmonary embolism (PE). This has an impact on the available choice of equipment, as the emphasis is on cardiac rather than peripheral work in most UK catheter labs.

The indications and contraindications for pulmonary angiography are listed in Table 6.7.

Table 6.7   Indications and contraindications for pulmonary angiography

Indications for pulmonary angiography	Pulmonary embolism
	Low probability V/Q scan with a high index of suspicion
	Intermediate probability V/Q scan with a high index of suspicion
	Pulmonary vasculitis
	Vascular malformation
Contraindications	
Absolute	None
Relative	Route specific
	Inferior vena cava filter
	Ileofemoral or superior vena cava thrombosis
	Pulmonary hypertension
	Right-sided valvular endocarditis

Potential complications

The overall complication rate during the PIOPED study [1], which undertook pulmonary angiography during suspected PE, was approximately 6.5 per cent. The complications are listed in Table 6.8.

Considerations for pulmonary angiography

ACCESS ROUTE

Pulmonary angiography can be achieved from almost any venous access route: femoral, subclavian, internal jugular or brachial veins. The choice of access site is important, depending on their clinical presentation. The patient with a PE following a long-term in-dwelling Hickman line is different from the patient with a deep-vein thrombosis (DVT) who presents with a PE. The access route for the former should not be via the superior vena cava (SVC), just as the latter should not be from the inferior vena cava (IVC). Access has been described in Chapter 3 for the brachial venous route and in Chapter 4 for the femoral route.

CATHETER CHOICE

The two main choices are balloon flotation catheters and pigtail catheters. Most catheter labs will carry a normal balloon catheter, with a distal thermistor suitable for right heart catheter to assess pressure, shunts and cardiac output by the modified Fick principle. They cannot be used for pulmonary angiography because they do not have multiple side holes and cannot tolerate the pressure generated by the power injector to get the contrast in a timely manner. We use a larger lumen 7F balloon- tipped catheter, but these are also end-hole catheters and are not designed for use with power injectors. There are other specifically

Table 6.8 Major complications of pulmonary angiography in the PIOPED study

Death	0.5%
Respiratory distress	0.4%
Renal failure	0.3%
Blood transfusion	0.2%
Urticaria	1.4%
Others	3.7%

designed balloon-tipped catheters with end and side holes for the purpose of pulmonary angiography.

Pigtail catheters are ideal, but the size of the curled segment really needs to be less than 1 cm to allow segmental angiography, and that can preclude some manufacturers' designs which are larger than this. They can be difficult to direct into the RV outflow tract and MPA from the RV, and then to direct into the right pulmonary artery (RPA).

TECHNIQUE

The first step is to position the catheter in the pulmonary artery, as described in the right heart catheterization section of this chapter. However, in contrast to our standard technique for right heart catheterization (i.e. getting to the pulmonary artery and performing saturation and pressure recordings on withdrawal), we recommend that the pressures should be recorded on the way in. A full haemodynamic assessment will enable other pathologies such as tamponade, cardiac restriction/constriction or left heart failure to be excluded, providing a catheter is also placed in the LV.

VIEWS AND ACQUISITION

Pulmonary angiograms are acquired in the posteroanterior (PA) view for both lungs, and the right anterior oblique (RAO) 45° view for the right lung and the left anterior oblique (LAO) 45° view for the left. The power injector should be set at 35–45 mL at a rate of 15–20 mL/s. It is best to acquire the lung, then wait for the left atrium to appear after 4–6 s; this second phase allows assessment of pulmonary vein anatomy, which is increasingly important as our electrophysiological colleagues start to ablate pulmonary veins for atrial fibrillation. It is also reasonable to acquire both oblique and PA views to reduce risk of angiographic signs being missed. This imparts a significant contrast load, unless a biplane lab is being used.

ANATOMY

The anatomy is discussed in Chapter 2.

Angiographic findings

The major findings include thrombus, dilated proximal pulmonary arteries, pulmonary arterial and venous stenosis and arteriovenous fistula.

THROMBUS

This is seen as an intraluminal filling defect. Although contrast may be seen partially passing the obstruction, albeit usually with ill-defined, hazy borders, it may be very difficult to see if the obstruction is complete and the truncated artery is short. There are ways of distinguishing between acute and chronic thromboembolism [2], but in practice this is very difficult, and usually dependent on the clinical picture. The major predictors of chronic pulmonary thromboembolic disease are:

- Pouching – collections of contrast within organized thrombus
- Webs/bands
- Abrupt tapering or scalloped walls
- Obstruction.

Realistically, PE should be diagnosed by V/Q scan or CT pulmonary angiography to avoid errors of interpretation, as our radiological colleagues see a lot more V/Q scans and CT pulmonary angiograms than we see pulmonary angiograms as cardiologists. However, in the patient with a raised troponin with ECG changes, who turns out to have essentially normal coronary arteries and normal LV function, it can occasionally be a useful investigation.

PULMONARY ARTERIAL AND VENOUS STENOSIS

The presence of a pulmonary artery stenosis may be associated with other congenital abnormalities such as Fallot's tetralogy, congenital aortic or pulmonary valvular stenosis, patent ductus arteriosus and truncus arteriosus. It is also commonly seen as a maladaptive vascular response to (partially) corrective surgery, such as Blalock shunts or Glenn procedures. It may also appear as an isolated finding, or as a response to chronic pulmonary infections. The pressure drop should be measured directly, as this may be severe despite mild angiographic appearances. However, bear in mind that a 6F catheter will take up space in the stenosis and cause some overestimation of the severity of the stenosis. With advances in interventional technique, cases of pulmonary arterial stenosis may be treated by balloon dilatation.

Pulmonary venous stenosis is uncommon, but likely to become more common as the number of pulmonary venous ablation procedures for AF increases.

ARTERIOVENOUS MALFORMATIONS

These are usually easy to identify, with rapid appearance of the malformation and premature appearance of contrast in the pulmonary venous system. Potentially they may be coiled. Usually this lies mostly in the province of interventional radiology, but may be tackled as a combined procedure between cardiologists and radiologists.

Renal angiography

Anatomy

The kidneys are located behind the peritoneum, on either side of the upper lumbar vertebrae. The left kidney usually sits slightly higher than the right. Both kidneys are located posteriorly and laterally to the aorta, so the renal arteries have to take a posterior oblique direction once they have arisen from the aorta. The consequence of this is that an oblique angiographic view is needed to adequately visualize the mid portion of each renal artery. The renal arteries arise at the level of the first lumbar vertebra, with the right renal artery crossing behind the IVC. Both renal arteries lie behind the corresponding renal vein. Coeliac and superior mesenteric arteries arise at T12 and L1 respectively. There may be a number of additional arteries supplying each kidney as well as the main renal artery, but in the main these still enter the kidney through the renal hilum. Occasionally, a polar artery may enter the superior or inferior renal pole directly. This has been shown in some historical studies in as many as 30 per cent of cases, when the extra vessel usually supplies the lower pole.

The role of angiography is in delineating the anatomy of the renal arteries prior to consideration of angioplasty and/or stenting of a focal stenosis. It is difficult to infer any assessment of function from angiographic pictures, other than microvascular flow from renal blush. Renal infarction will show up as a wedge-shaped perfusion defect if it is acute.

Renal angiography is highly unlikely to occur in the cardiac centre as an isolated procedure, and therefore the calibre of the vascular sheath is usually determined by lab policy for routine coronary angiography. There is an ongoing argument between radiologists and cardiologists regarding the ownership of renal angiography and the role of the technique performed in patients having their coronary arteries studied. Nevertheless, in the presence of established coronary artery disease, significant atherosclerotic renovascular disease will occur in approximately 20 per cent of cases, and the figure may be higher than this in hypertensive patients with angiographic disease. This justifies the extra time and the extra contrast. Improvement following renal angioplasty may stabilize renal function, and may also improve hypertension control and clinical outcome.

Typically, the cardiac phase of the procedure is performed first, followed by the renal phase, as the late-phase nephrogram may help to identify kidney location.

Technique

Initial interrogation of renal anatomy would normally involve a flush aortogram using a pigtail catheter, usually positioned with the pigtail one vertebral level above the ostium of the renal artery at T12/L1. High flow rates are required, with 40–50 mL of contrast, delivered at 15–20 mL/min, as suboptimal injection rates will lead to missed ostial disease. If biplane angiograpy is available, then two runs should be performed, the first in monoplane as a PA view, the second as a biplane RAO 25° LAO 25°. This should provide enough information about the ostium and the body of the renal arteries, areas that are amenable to intervention. Occasionally the course of the artery is abnormal and the views may need to be changed.

Selective angiography may be required if adequate definition is not obtained by the flush aortogram. Catheter selection for selective renal angiography is usually a simple process, and it is rarely necessary to resort to specific radiographic catheters. All renal arteries can usually be selectively engaged with either a Judkins R4 or an internal mammary catheter. If difficulties are experienced with these choices then a Williams catheter may be needed. Accessory renal arteries need particular care, as they may be easily missed, so it is important to make sure that perfusion to all parts of the kidney is visualized.

It is prudent to keep acquiring until the nephrogram and then the late phase of renal venous flow is clearly seen. This may help in diagnosis of renal infarct, renal vein thrombosis, etc.

Angiographic findings

There are two major disease entities affecting the renal arteries: atherosclerotic disease and fibromuscular dysplasia.

ATHEROSCLEROTIC RENOVASCULAR DISEASE

Classical atherosclerotic plaque tends to affect the perirenal aorta, the renal artery ostium and the proximal third of the renal artery. It has the same risk factors as atherosclerotic disease anywhere: diabetes, smoking, hypertension, etc. It is a progressive disease, and is a significant cause for chronic renal failure and renal replacement therapy.

The angiographic appearance is typical of plaque disease and, when coupled with the location of the disease, gives the diagnosis. Treatment is possible with percutaneous intervention (PCI), but patient selection is the key factor, as PCI may provoke renal failure due to distal embolization of plaque material. Renal intervention has been demonstrated to prevent deterioration in renal function and also to reduce antihypertensive drug requirements in carefully selected patients.

FIBROMUSCULAR DYSPLASIA

This condition predominantly occurs in younger female patients (15–50 years) and may represent about 10 per cent of renovascular hypertension cases. It is characterized by a classical angiographic appearance – the 'string of beads' – which typically affects the mid to distal portion of the coronary artery, although the histological appearance is less pathognomonic and is one of an abnormal medial layer of elastic tissue. It may well coexist with atherosclerotic renovascular disease.

Fibromuscular dysplasia is eminently treatable by balloon angioplasty, with stenting being reserved for bale-out situation with procedural dissection.

References

1. Stein PD, Athanasoulis C, Alavi A *et al.* Complications and validity of pulmonary angiography in acute pulmonary embolism. *Circulation* 1992; **85:** 462–468.
2. Auger WR, Fedullo PF, Moser KM *et al.* Chronic major-vessel thromboembolic pulmonary artery obstruction: appearance at angiography. *Radiology* 1992; **182:** 393–398.

Complications of cardiac catheterization

7

The overall rate of major complications for cardiac catheterization runs at between 1 per cent and 2 per cent. However, the likelihood of major complications increases significantly with the severity of the underlying cardiac and non-cardiac disease. Patients with both valvular and coronary artery disease are more likely to sustain a complication than patients with isolated coronary artery disease. Similarly, additional comorbidities also increase the overall risk of the procedure. For example, any of the following will suggest a higher risk at cardiac catheterization:

- Diabetes
- Age >80
- Low body mass index (BMI) <25

- High BMI >35
- Female sex
- Peripheral vascular disease.

Prudent precautions

The following precautions are advisable:

1. Secure intravenous access in all patients. Hypotension because of a vagal reaction to catheterization can be rapid and profound. A 21 g intravenous cannula should be present in all patients who undergo catheter lab procedures.
2. Make sure that atropine is readily available.
3. Ensure a defibrillator is readily available, preferably with self-adhesive pads that can attach to the patient.
4. Ensure that an intra-aortic balloon pump is readily accessible, and the appropriate expertise for timely insertion is available.

Most procedures in the catheter lab are, however, relatively straightforward and as access routes and the quality and size of equipment improves, complication rates are likely to be reduced further. When problems do occur they may be sudden and progress rapidly; they can also be fatal. It is incumbent on any person in the lab to be able to recognize and deal with emergencies in a calm and efficient manner. The main complications seen are listed in Table 7.1.

Contrast reactions

General guidelines for the diagnosis and treatment of contrast reactions have been published elsewhere [1,2]. Most treatment protocols are based on radiological practice, but the principles equally apply to the cardiac catheter lab. Indeed in the catheter lab we have the advantage of online ECG and arterial pressure monitoring and venous access, which may not be present or easily accessible in the radiology lab.

Mild contrast reactions are common, although the data are now quite old and relate to hypertonic contrast media. The Registry of the Society for Angiography and Intervention suggest a total adverse event rate of approximately 8 per cent. This equates to 1 in 12 patients, which

Table 7.1 Major complications of cardiac catheterization

Immediate reactions	
Contrast reactions	
Arrhythmia	Bradycardia
	Atrial fibrillation
	Ventricular tachycardia
	Ventricular fibrillation
Hypotension	Haemorrhage
	Vagal reaction
Tamponade	
Coronary artery complications	Dissection
	Air embolism
	Spasm
Death	
Myocardial infarction	
Stroke	
Cannulation site complications	Haematoma
	False aneurysm
	Arteriovenous fistula
	Retrograde dissection
Delayed reactions	
Radiodermatitis	
Angiography associated renal dysfunction	
Contrast nephropathy	
Atheroembolic renal dysfunction	

means that, in real terms, we are likely to see some sort of reaction to contrast in every other catheter list. Severe systemic reactions are much less common and occur in one in every 500 cases, with a fatality rate of one in 55 000.

There are two main types of contrast reaction:

- Anaphylactoid
- Chemotoxic.

Anaphylactoid reactions

There is often confusion about the nature of contrast reactions, which are anaphylactoid not anaphylactic, although the presentation is the same and the distinction in the catheter lab largely academic. Anaphylaxis is an immunoglobulin E (IgE)-mediated hypersensitivity reaction, requiring prior sensitization to an antigen. Once sensitized, further exposure will cause the generation of the antibody–antigen complex, which binds to mast cells, stimulating histamine release amongst other vasoactive agents. It is therefore an immune-mediated reaction, dependent on antibody formation, which contrasts with an anaphylactoid reaction.

The pathophysiological background to anaphylactoid reactions, on the other hand, is not well understood although the final pathway is also mast cell degranulation and the consequent widespread release of histamine. Anaphylactoid reactions have also been shown variously to activate the complement system both directly and indirectly by anaphylatoxins. There is also some evidence of alteration of the coagulation and fibrinolytic pathways.

In both cases histamine is the major contributor to systemic and local reactions. Histamine can either come from basophils or mast cells and exerts its actions via H_1 and H_2 receptors. H_1 receptors mediate what we would intuitively know as 'allergic' phenomena (i.e. changes in vascular permeability, bronchospasm and vasodilatation). However, the H_2 receptor also contributes to increased vascular permeability and vasodilatation. Data certainly suggest that H_1 mediates the majority of the anaphylactoid reaction but that H_2 makes a sizeable contribution and that treatment with antagonists of both are at least additive and probably synergistic.

Chemotoxic effects

Contrast media also produce a spectrum of chemotoxic effects, which are primarily due to their hyperosmolarity, viscosity and calcium-binding properties. The incidence has reduced with the use of low-osmolarity contrast media. Mild vasodilatory reactions such as the sensation of heat/burning on left ventriculography pass within 30 seconds, but can be disturbing. Severe reactions are difficult to separate from anaphylactoid reactions and should probably be managed similarly. The electrophysiological changes of ST–T wave changes, bradycardia, PR and QT prolongation are usually transitory, but atrioventricular (AV) block can be precipitated. Its management is discussed later in the chapter. Depression in myocardial function may be seen, although this usually only causes symptoms if it is the final insult for a struggling heart. The management of contrast-induced chemotoxic reactions is summarized in Table 7.2.

Table 7.2 Management of contrast-induced chemotoxic reactions

Chemotoxicity reaction	Management
Arteriolar vasodilatation – manifesting as a sensation of heat, hypotension	**Mild reaction**
	No action necessary
	Moderate reaction
	Intravenous (i.v.) fluids
	Severe reaction
	Rapid i.v. fluid replacement
	Epinephrine 0.3 mg subcutaneously every 15 min – if unresponsive
	Epinephrine 10 µg bolus i.v. followed by infusion 1–4 µg/min
ECG changes	**Severe reaction** (severe bradycardia/complete heart block)
	Atropine 600 µg repeated up to 3 times
	Temporary venous pacing
Nausea/vomiting	i.v. antiemetics
Depression of myocardial function	
Manifesting as hypotension	**Moderate/severe reaction**
	Angiographer needs to make decision about treatment modality
	i.v. inotropic support
	Intra-aortic balloon pump (IABP)
	Urgent revascularization
Manifesting as pulmonary oedema	**Moderate/severe reaction**
	Angiographer needs to make decision about treatment modality
	i.v. glyceryl trinitrate (GTN)
	IABP
	i.v. diuretic

i.v., intravenous.

Recognition

The patient will often report mild symptoms initially. The difficulty is that the operator does not know whether this is a harbinger for a more severe reaction or will remain a mild reaction (Figure 7.1). The main clinical scenarios are listed in Table 7.3.

The differential diagnosis is also quite wide (Table 7.4).

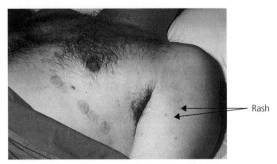

Figure 7.1   Mild contrast reaction: pruritic rash.

Table 7.3 The clinical presentation of mild, moderate and major contrast reactions

Minor reaction	Moderate reaction	Major reaction
Urticaria (limited)	Urticaria (widespread)	Shock
Pruritus	Angioedema	Respiratory arrest
Erythema	Laryngeal oedema	Cardiac arrest
	Bronchospasm	

Table 7.4 The differential diagnosis of contrast reactions

Cardiac	Non-cardiac
Vasovagal reactions	Hypovolaemia
Cardiogenic shock	Drug-related effects or reactions
Right ventricular infarction	Sepsis
Cardiac tamponade	
Cardiac rupture	

Prevention

There are three main categories of patients at risk:

- The patient with a prior anaphylactoid reaction
- The allergic patient
- The biphasic reaction.

PRIOR ANAPHYLACTOID REACTION

Patients with prior contrast reaction are at increased risk of subsequent contrast reaction, but it is not always predictable. A patient can have been exposed to contrast previously without ill-effect and yet have a life-threatening event on the next exposure. Conversely, a life-threatening event may not be followed by any reaction at all. However, those with a previous reaction have a 16–44 per cent incidence of another reaction with subsequent exposure to contrast media [3].

It is important to note that prophylaxis is not completely protective, and the lab must still be vigilant and prepared for a serious reaction.

THE ALLERGIC PATIENT

The second category at high risk is the patient with atopy/asthma, who may be twice as likely to develop a contrast reaction [5]. Food allergies have no impact [5].

THE BIPHASIC REACTION

The final group at risk is those who have had a contrast reaction that has been effectively treated, who go on to have a further reaction after discharge without further exposure to contrast. The first 48 hours are important for this and although there are no randomized trial data to support practice guidelines, patients who have a contrast reaction should be treated with ongoing oral steroids for a further 48 hours following the index event and preferably monitored in hospital overnight, unless the reaction is mild.

Prevention

PHARMACOLOGICAL PRETREATMENT

There are two mechanisms of drug prophylaxis – steroids and histamine antagonists. The current recommendation of the Society for Angiography and Intervention is to pretreat with 50 mg of prednisone (prednisalone) orally at 13, 7 and 1 hours and give diphenhydramine 50 mg orally 1 hour before the planned procedure. This was shown to be effective in reducing recurrent events [1].

Alternative strategies include prescribing 30 mg of prednisone twice daily and chlorpheniramine 10 mg three times a day for 48 hours before and after the case. H_2 antagonists are available in the catheter lab as intravenous preparations but are reserved for severe reactions.

In the emergency situation, where a patient with a previous contrast reaction presents for urgent angiography, then 200 mg hydrocortisone plus intravenous H_1 antagonist should be given as soon as possible, unless the coronary procedure can be delayed. We prefer chlorpheniramine (Piriton) to promethazine (Phenergan) as our experience suggests that it causes less periprocedural confusion and paradoxical agitation.

CHOICE OF CONTRAST AGENTS

Previously there was debate about the use of newer non-ionic/low-osmolar contrast media versus the older, more established media such as urograffin. There appear to be fewer contrast reactions [1], but not all agree this reduction was worth the cost differential [6]. Nevertheless, most centres now use non-ionic media.

Treatment

The treatment options for the main presenting scenarios of an anaphylactoid contrast reaction are summarized in Table 7.5.

Arrhythmia

Arrhythmias are common in the catheter lab, either as a pre-existing condition or as a complication of the procedure. A comprehensive overview of arrhythmia management is outside the scope of this book, and is covered extensively elsewhere. Here we will limit ourselves to abnormalities of rhythm that complicate diagnostic angiography, ranging from common accompaniments such as benign ventricular extrasystoles caused by catheter contact with left ventricular wall, to the immediate life-threatening ventricular fibrillation caused by the inadvertent injection of contrast down a small vessel or contrast stasis.

It goes without saying that it is incumbent on all laboratory personnel to watch the physiology monitor in the catheter lab. The occurrence of any arrhythmia should be immediately highlighted to the cardiologist. The laboratory should be equipped with a defibrillator capable of administering a series of rapid DC countershocks that can be synchronous or asynchronous. Temporary pacing wires, appropriate connectors and a functioning pacing box should be immediately to hand, as

Table 7.5 Management of anaphylactoid contrast reactions

General treatment (to all patients)	**Mild/moderate**
	200 mg i.v. hydrocortisone
	12.5–25 mg i.v. promethazine or 10–20 mg chlorpheniramine
	Severe
	As above plus i.v. ranitidine 50 mg/cimetidine 300 mg
Urticaria	**Mild/moderate**
	200 mg i.v. hydrocortisone
	12.5–25 mg i.v. promethazine or 10–20 mg chlorpheniramine
	Severe
	As above plus i.v. ranitidine 50 mg/cimetidine 300 mg
Bronchospasm	O_2 via face mask
	Mild
	Salbutamol 200 µg via metered dose inhaler
	Moderate
	Salbutamol or 5 mg via nebulizer ±ipratropium bromide 500 µg nebulized
	12.5–25 mg i.v. promethazine or 10–20 mg chlorpheniramine
	Epinephrine 0.3 mg s.c. every 15 min
	Severe
	Salbutamol or 5 mg via nebulizer ±ipratropium bromide 500 µg nebulized
	Epinephrine 10 µg bolus i.v. followed by infusion 1–4 µg/min
	i.v. ranitidine 50 mg/cimetidine 300 mg
Facial and/or laryngeal oedema	**Mild/moderate**
	O_2 via face mask
	200 mg i.v. hydrocortisone
	12.5–25 mg i.v. promethazine or 10–20 mg chlorpheniramine
	Severe
	As above plus rapid anaesthetic assessment
	Epinephrine 0.3 mg s.c. every 15 min – if unresponsive
	Epinephrine 10 µg bolus i.v. followed by infusion 1–4 µg/min
	i.v. ranitidine 50 mg/cimetidine 300 mg
Hypotension/ shock	O_2 via face mask
	Large volume of i.v. fluids (1–3 L in first hour)
	200 mg i.v. hydrocortisone
	12.5–25 mg i.v. promethazine or 10–20 mg chlorpheniramine
	i.v. ranitidine 50 mg/cimetidine 300 mg
	Epinephrine 0.3 mg s.c. every 15 min – if unresponsive
	Epinephrine 10 µg bolus i.v. followed by infusion 1–4 µg/min
	Advanced cardiac life support
	Phenylephrine may have a role as a peripheral arteriolar vasoconstrictor injected into the peripheral vasculature in 200–300 µg aliquots

i.v., intravenous.

should a full range of drugs. Nursing personnel should be familiar with making up all the drugs in the lab and there should never be a situation where the nurse has to leave the room to get advice on how to make up/administer an emergency drug. All key catheter laboratory staff should hold an up-to-date Advanced Life Support (ALS) certificate, including the operator, run nurse, physiology technician and radiographer. The role of each member of staff in the catheter lab during a cardiac arrest should be predetermined and clearly understood.

Atrial arrhythmias

ATRIAL EXTRASYSTOLES

Atrial extrasystoles are common when manipulating catheters in the right atrium and need no specific treatment. The risk is that they may degenerate further into atrial fibrillation (AF) or atrial flutter.

ATRIAL FIBRILLATION

AF is generally benign during the process of coronary catheterization, and often spontaneously cardioverts back to sinus rhythm during or immediately after the procedure. However, some patients are at risk of sudden haemodynamic decompensation, when sinus rhythm degenerates to AF with a rapid ventricular rate: hypertrophic obstructive cardiomyopathy, poor left ventricular function or critical aortic and mitral stenosis. The loss of the atrial contribution to left ventricle filling can reduce cardiac output by as much as 30 per cent.

Initial management is directed at rate control to allow the completion of the procedure. This can be achieved with an intravenous preparation of beta-blockers or rate-limiting calcium channel blockers. The intravenous doses are listed in Chapter 8. Caution is necessary before intravenous administration of AV nodal blocking agents in subjects already receiving AV nodal blocking agents of a different class (i.e. intravenous beta-blockers in patients taking verapamil or diltiazem). Knowledge of pre-existing medication, therefore, is important to avoid inadvertent complete heart block.

Cardioversion may be achieved in three ways. If there is haemodynamic compromise then a synchronized external DC shock should be applied at 50 J for flutter or 100 J for AF. This should be accompanied by intravenous administration of an anxiolytic such as diazepam or midazolam for both the anxiety relief and amnesic properties. The second mechanism is rapid atrial pacing. If the right heart has been accessed, a short 15 second burst of rapid atrial pacing (300–400 beats per minute) may achieve sinus rhythm. The final mechanism is chemical cardioversion. In the USA agents such as quinidine or procainamide are commonly used, but in the UK flecainide or amiodarone are more likely. The bolus should be given in the lab and the infusion should be continued in the recovery area. The arterial sheath should remain *in situ* to allow arterial pressure monitoring. Flecainide has received a bad press because of the CAST study, where it was used to suppress ventricular ectopy postmyocardial infarction [7]. The single dose in the catheter lab to cardiovert AF, even in the presence of coronary artery disease, is entirely different.

Ventricular arrhythmia

VENTRICULAR EXTRASYSTOLES

Ventricular extrasystoles are common when manipulating catheters in the left and right ventricles. Therefore careful and smooth passage of right heart and pigtail catheters is desirable, but not always possible. A sudden increase in ectopic activity is an indicator that the catheter is not in an ideal position and should be moved. This is particularly relevant with positioning the pigtail catheter in the left ventricular cavity.

VENTRICULAR TACHYCARDIA AND FIBRILLATION

Ventricular tachycardia (VT) can be provoked in up to 30 per cent of right heart catheter investigations, being sustained in 3 per cent and degenerating into ventricular fibrillation (VF) in 0.7 per cent [8]. More commonly, non-sustained VT is seen with malpositioning of the left ventricular pigtail catheter, or too forceful an injection or too large a contrast volume injected into the LV cavity.

However, VF is more likely to be due to contrast injection, particularly into the right coronary or circumflex arteries. This was very problematical when contrast media were ionic and hyperosmolar, but now the incidence of VT and VF has dropped to 0.4 per cent in the most recent Society for Angiography Registry [9]. The problem seems to occur when contrast remains static within the coronary artery and inflow is obstructed, either with selective engagement of a sub-branch (classically the conus branch), overengagement or because of the presence of an ostial lesion. If pressure damping occurs, then contrast should not be injected, or should be injected very cautiously. When the catheter has been repositioned and there is no pressure damping a cautious injection is made. Intracoronary glyceryl trinitrate (GTN) may be helpful in relieving spasm.

The management of non-sustained VT centres on removing the precipitant and may well mean nothing more than repositioning a catheter. However multiple episodes, especially if symptomatic may warrant treatment. Lignocaine (lidocaine) or amiodarone are potential choices, but the latter is preferred if LV function is impaired. Electrolytes (Mg^{2+} and K^+) should be rechecked.

Sustained VT is treated initially by removing any obvious precipitant, such as a malpositioned catheter. If there is haemodynamic compromise immediate non-synchronized DC countershock must be administered, even if the patient remains conscious. This avoids the need for cardiopulmonary resuscitation (CPR) and the concomitant risk of desterilization of the surgical field. It can be followed by an intravenous benzodiazepine-based sedative, for the associated amnesic properties of this class of drug.

If there is no haemodynamic compromise there are three alternatives: pharmacological termination with lignocaine (lidocaine) or amiodarone, pacing-mediated termination, or DC countershock. One strategy is to give 100 mg of lignocaine (lidocaine) if LV function is normal or amiodarone 300 mg intravenous if not, and give it a minute to work; meanwhile place a 5 or 6F sheath in the right femoral vein (RFV) and pass a 5F temporary pacing wire to the right ventricle (RV) apex. Even if the lignocaine (lidocaine) works, you now have venous access to utilize antitachycardia pacing strategies if necessary. If both fail, or the patient becomes unstable, then non-synchronized DC countershock is indicated.

TEMPORARY ANTITACHYCARDIA PACING

A temporary pacing wire may be positioned in the RV apex and attempts made to terminate by pacing. Once the temporary pacing catheter is in the RV apex, the VT rate is assessed. If the rate is <150 bpm, then an attempt at underdrive pacing can be attempted. VT with rates higher than this rarely terminate with this method. A rate 10–20 per cent slower than the tachycardia is chosen and asynchronous pacing maintained for 30 seconds. If this fails to entrain the VT then attempt overdrive pace termination next.

If the rate is >150 bpm or underdrive pacing has failed, then an attempt at overdrive pacing is warranted. In this situation a rate 20–30 per cent faster than the tachycardia is chosen. A burst of pacing is introduced and once entrainment occurs – where each pacing spike is associated with a QRS complex – then the pacing is abruptly terminated. The risk with this strategy is that overdrive pacing can accelerate VT, turning a haemodynamically stable tachycardia into an unstable one or that is may cause degeneration into VF. Failure of termination or degradation of the tachycardia is an indication for the immediate administration of a non-synchronized DC countershock.

DC COUNTERSHOCK

This is usually administered by either the physiology technician, radiographer or circulating/run nurse according to local practice. If the patient is very unstable (i.e. unconscious or presyncopal) then an immediate shock is necessary. However, if the rhythm is being tolerated, it is not unreasonable to give a small dose of an intravenous anxiolytic pre shock, and an opiate analgesia post shock. Failure of cardioversion in the context of haemodynamic instability requires CPR and the initiation of standard VT ALS protocols and the summoning of senior help.

If the patient is stable and other methods of termination have failed then sedation may be administered pre shock. If an anaesthetist is available immediately then it is appropriate to use their skills; otherwise give a dose of midazolam, which can be titrated up to achieve a state where the conscious level is appropriately depressed. They may then be cardioverted in the lab. Once stable, complete the procedure.

CONSCIOUS SEDATION

Conscious sedation protocols need to be developed in-house. Ideally, the operator induces a depressed level of consciousness, in which a patient can maintain a patent airway independently and continuously and can be aroused by physical stimuli. Patients in this state cannot hold a conversation, but should be able to respond to commands. It is important to recognize that patients can sometimes enter a state of deep sedation unexpectedly. In this state the patient is not easily aroused and there may be partial or complete loss of protective reflexes, including the inability to consistently maintain a patent airway independently and the inability to respond purposefully to physical stimulation or verbal commands.

Consequently it is prudent to have an oxygen delivery system, appropriate airway management equipment (e.g. masks, oral airways, endotracheal tubes and laryngoscopes) and suction equipment to hand. There also needs to be appropriate monitoring of oxygenation (pulse oximeter), arterial pressure and heart rate. Perhaps more importantly there needs to be a resuscitation trolley and the ability to call for more senior assistance. The appropriate pharmacologic antagonists, including naloxone and flumazenil, should be immediately available.

Bradycardia

Bradycardias are common during coronary procedures, although the incidence is dropping as the use of non-ionic low osmolar contrast becomes the norm.

Transient bradycardia may occur during injection of right coronary or dominant circumflex arteries. This may manifest as a sinus bradycardia, ventricular standstill or even asystole. It is usually transient, and rhythm returns to normal as contrast clears. It can be treated by asking the patient to cough vigorously, which stimulates ventricular extrasystoles and can maintain limited cardiac output for a short period. In addition it also helps to clear contrast from the coronary artery. If symptoms are more prolonged then an alternative cause needs to be sought.

VASOVAGAL REACTIONS

These are accompanied by hypotension, nausea, sweating and yawning. Bradycardia is often a prominent feature. Vagal reactions occur in 3 per cent of cases and most adverse vasovagal reactions (80 per cent) occur during vascular access and 16 per cent during sheath removal. Vasovagal reactions are triggered by pain, anxiety and exacerbated by hypovolaemia.

Judicious local analgesia may be very helpful, especially in radial procedures early in the learning curve. Routine premedication with an anxiolytic is usually unnecessary. Intravenous atropine is the mainstay of therapy (0.3–1.2 mg), associated with volume expansion, by both raising the legs and intravenous fluid infusion. If these measures fail and bradycardia remains an issue, then temporary pacing is needed. If the rate increases, but pressure remains low, then inotropic support is necessary with adrenaline, dobutamine, dopamine or intra-aortic balloon pumping. Some patients, such as those with severe aortic stenosis, are particularly at risk of a catastophic decompensation if the vagal reaction is not treated promptly.

BUNDLE BRANCH AND ATRIOVENTRICULAR BLOCK

There are a few circumstances where pre-existing bundle branch block can cause trouble. Catheter manipulation in the RV outflow tract in the presence of left bundle branch block (LBBB) can provoke transitory complete block, because of the compact nature of the right bundle. When complete AV block occurs, the risk of impending cardiovascular collapse needs to be assessed. If the rate is >45 bpm and ventricular escape complexes are narrow and blood pressure is being maintained with a systolic pressure greater than 100 mmHg, then it most likely will be well tolerated and only conservative therapy is required. However, if the rate is slow, the complexes broad and pressure falling, then the following steps should be taken:

1. Administer atropine 0.6 mg (may not help, but unlikely to do harm).
2. Ask the patient to cough regularly (1 per second).
3. Give adrenaline 1–2 μg intracoronary slowly or 10 μg intravenously slowly.
4. Apply transcutaneous pacing until temporary transvenous pacing wire can be inserted.

Hypotension

Hypotension is common in the catheter lab and is usually due to one or a combination of the following:

- Hypovolaemia
- Vasodilatation
- Tamponade
- Impaired LV function
- Rarely: acute valvular regurgitation.

Hypovolaemia

Hypovolaemia is a common occurrence, because patients are often starved overnight prior to entering the catheterization lab. This may be exacerbated by a number of factors, including intravascular depletion due to concomitant diuretic administration, the duration of the procedure causing dehydration or a contrast-induced diuresis. All are simply treated with an infusion of 0.9 per cent saline.

Hypovolaemia can also be seen following a vascular injury associated with haemorrhage. The most common is the femoral puncture site, either because of leakage around the sheath, multiple punctures, damage to other vessels or too high a puncture leading to retroperitoneal bleeding. The groin puncture site should be always be checked during an episode of hypotension. The management of femoral complications is discussed in Chapter 4. If no obvious bleeding source or haematoma is seen, an urgent estimation of the haemoglobin level should be sought, and a retroperitoneal haematoma considered as a potential cause.

Vasodilatation

Vasodilatation may be part of a vasovagal syndrome, accompanied by the diagnostic clues of bradycardia, yawning and sweating. Treatment is with atropine 0.3–1.2 mg intravenously and volume replacement with 0.9 per cent saline.

However, there is always the possibility of a contrast reaction, which should be considered in a case of unexplained hypotension.

Failure of prompt correction of hypotension suggests the need for a right heart catheter to assess filling pressures. High filling pressures suggest a cardiac cause such as cardiac tamponade or myocardial dysfunction, whereas low filling pressures suggest intravascular volume depletion or vasodilatation. A point of interest is that the pulmonary artery normally has a saturation in the region of 70 per cent. In certain cases of hypotension such as a contrast reaction, sepsis or an idiosyncratic drug reaction, the resulting massive vasodilatation causes arteriovenous shunting and a rise in P_AO_2 saturation.

Cardiac tamponade

Cardiac perforation is related to procedures in which stiffer catheters are used: procedures involving septal puncture such as electrophysiological procedures, endomyocardial biopsy, balloon valvuloplasty and temporary pacing catheters. The incidence appears to be higher in elderly women. Care should be exercised in the manipulation of stiff catheters.

When perforation occurs, the first signs tend to be due to vagal stimulation from blood irritating the pericardium and may manifest as hypotension and bradycardia. The arterial pressure trace may show paradox, where the pulse pressure falls >10 mmHg with inspiration.

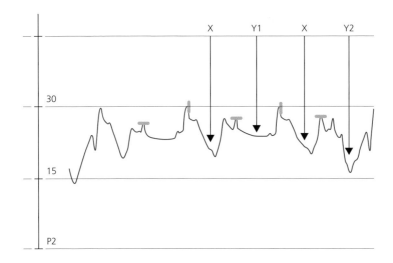

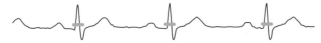

Figure 7.2 Right atrial pressure in cardiac tamponade. Raised pressure is seen throughout the trace. The *y* descent is absent (*y*1), but returns with aspiration (*y*2). (Trace is edited.)

If a right heart catheter is in the venous system the trace will show elevation of the right heart pressure and a loss of the *y* descent (Figure 7.2). If the situation is developing slowly, then transthoracic echocardiography is necessary to confirm the diagnosis.

However, if the patient is haemodynamically unstable with hypotension, arterial paradox plus or minus right heart evidence of tamponade then immediate pericardiocentesis should be performed. The pericardiocentesis kit should be available immediately, and the operator should be familiar with the kit that is used locally.

Some centres give small doses of heparin before diagnostic cases, a practice more commonly seen in the USA. In this situation it is prudent to aspirate to dryness if possible and then reverse the systemic heparinization with protamine sulphate. Reversing too early has the theoretical risk of causing blood to clot within the pericardial sac, making aspiration difficult. Increasingly effective antiplatelet treatment of non-ST elevation myocardial infarction with clopidogrel and glycoprotein (GP) IIb–IIIa inhibitors may make haemostasis more difficult. Most cardiac perforations self-seal. In a Mayo Clinic series cardiac perforation occurred in 0.08 per cent of overall catheter laboratory cases, but in only 0.006 per cent of cardiac catheterizations. Of those who had tamponade, over 80 per cent settled with pericardiocentesis alone, the rest required surgery [10].

Left ventricular and acute valvular dysfunction

Complications causing acute ischaemia or valve damage severe enough to cause hypotension are rare during diagnostic procedures.

Myocardial ischaemia (MI) and/or infarction may occur for a number of reasons, including abrupt occlusion and intimal dissection. The incidence of catheter-related ischaemia/MI increases with the following factors:

- Severity of disease
- Left main stem disease
- Three-vessel disease
- Ostial disease
- Recent acute coronary syndrome
- Diabetes mellitus.

ABRUPT OCCLUSION

This may be related to a number of causes, but commonly it is due to contrast-mediated platelet aggregation in a critically narrowed coronary artery or dissection. Because non-ionic, low-osmolar contrast is viscous, it may only pass through critical segments slowly. Platelet activation occurs with the accompanying stasis, creating a prothrombotic environment. This usually takes a little time, and often happens after the catheter has been withdrawn.

For example, a critical left main stem is identified and after a limited number of views, the catheter is disengaged and the right coronary views are acquired. After angiography, the patient begins to develop chest pain, hypotension and left-sided ECG changes. When the left coronary artery is re-engaged, the left main has occluded. The only option is revascularization. Supportive treatment with O_2, inotropes and a balloon pump are bridges to the definitive treatment, whether this be percutaneous intervention (PCI) or coronary artery bypass grafting (CABG).

CORONARY DISSECTION

Coronary dissection arises from instrumentation of the coronary artery. Dissection flaps are seen in the left main stem, right coronary ostium and first segments of the left anterior descending (LAD), circumflex and right coronary artery (RCA) if the catheter has been overengaged. The left main stem and RCA ostium are prone to dissection if a catheter is chosen that does not sit coaxially to the artery, increasing the risk of raising dissection flap and injecting contrast subintimally. Occasionally, localized coronary dissections can track backwards into the aortic root, or forwards down the coronary arteries. Dissections are recognized by the new appearance of a double lumen, a persistant 'cap' of contrast or a localized filling defect (Figures 7.3, 7.4 and 5.34).

A separate entity is spontaneous coronary dissection, which tends to occur in a younger population. There may be associations with physical stress, pregnancy and cocaine abuse.

Treatment is usually by revascularization, whether this is PCI or CABG. The presence of haemodynamic instability means that O_2, inotropic support and a balloon pump should be considered. The advice of a senior interventional colleague is a sensible precaution, as the left main could be stented as a definitive treatment or as a bridge to CABG.

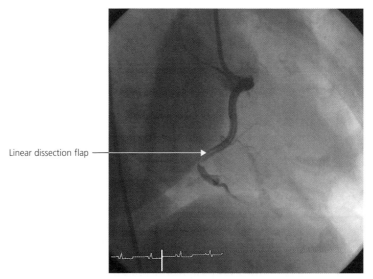

Linear dissection flap

Figure 7.3   Dissection of right coronary artery.

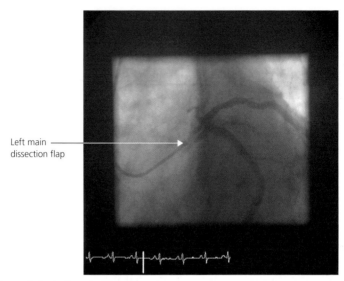

Left main
dissection flap

Figure 7.4 Left main dissection.

Similarly, surgical colleagues will appreciate knowing sooner rather than later that a candidate for an operative intervention is heading their way.

ACUTE VALVULAR DAMAGE

This is uncommon, but perforation of aortic valves or damage of mitral subvalvular apparatus may be caused by a pigtail catheter. The only treatment is surgical correction. Balloon pumps cannot be used as a supportive treatment in acute aortic regurgitation, as they will increase the regurgitant fraction.

Death, myocardial infarction and stroke

Death

There has been a significant decline in the risk of death from diagnostic cardiac catheterization. The last Society for Cardiac Angiography and Interventions (SCA&I) data set showed a risk of death in left main stem disease of 0.86 per cent and single vessel disease of 0.03 per cent [9]. In a more recent data set from the UK, in over 2000 cardiac catheterizations

Table 7.6 Predictors of death

Age	<1 year and >60 years
Functional class	Class IV have ×10 risk of death compared with classes I–II
Disease severity	Left main stem disease has a ×10 increased risk
Valvular disease	Concomitant valve disease increases risk of death
Left ventricular dysfunction	Ejection fraction (EF) <30% is associated with ×10 mortality risk compared with EF >50%
Severe co-morbidities	The following all increase risk of death: renal impairment, diabetes, peripheral vascular disease, chronic obstructive pulmonary disease

Adapted from Baim Donald S and Grossman William (eds). *Grossman's Cardiac Catheterization, Angiography, and Intervention*, 6th edn. Philadelphia: Lippincott Williams & Wilkins, 2000, p. 37.

there were only two deaths, both with left main stem disease [11]. Nevertheless, certain patient characteristics predict death (Table 7.6).

The implication of these data is that left main stem disease is an important risk factor for an adverse outcome from diagnostic procedures. Therefore the first views should always provide adequate diagnostic information about the left main stem. Taking more views than necessary may increase risk. In order to minimize the risk of death, patients with potential left main stem disease, diabetes, renal failure and impaired left ventricular function should be as haemodynamically stable as possible. If the patient is not stable and the case is not urgent it is prudent to postpone the case to improve the patient's clinical status.

Myocardial infarction

MI was reported to occur in 0.05 per cent of diagnostic cases in the early 1990s [9] and in a more recent UK series of 2000 patients the occurrence was 0.001 per cent [11]. In these reports there were key patient and technique-based markers for higher risk of MI, including the severity of coronary disease (3 times increased risk in extensive disease), the presence of an acute coronary syndrome, diabetes and catheter complications such as dissection.

It is not routine to check a creatine kinase MB (CK-MB) or troponin level following uncomplicated diagnostic catheterization, so the incidence of asymptomatic non-ST elevation MI is unknown. The MIs that are picked up are likely to have been associated with ST segment changes or chest pain. The occurrence of either demands prompt action.

MANAGEMENT OF AN IN-LABORATORY MYOCARDIAL INFARCTION

The causes of MI in the lab are:

- Thrombus progression in acute coronary syndrome
- Abrupt closure – contrast viscosity, reduced coronary flow or air embolism
- Dissection.

The first steps of management are universal: oxygen, intravenous fluid and opiate analgesia. The next step is to identify the cause and the likely mechanism of recovery. This is likely to demand the presence of senior colleagues and they should be summoned sooner rather than later.

The situation may be recoverable with PCI, and if available on site then this should take place immediately. The catheter laboratory's normal procedures should then be activated. The patient should be given aspirin and clopidogrel orally. If the patient is not receiving chronic oral antiplatelet therapy then 300 mg of soluble aspirin and 600 mg of clopidogrel should be administered to aid rapid onset of action. The dose of heparin and use of GP IIb–IIIa inhibitors is at the interventional cardiologist's discretion. If PCI is not available on site or surgery is necessary, then a balloon pump should be inserted, and transfer arranged urgently.

If hypotension is present, but no clinical heart failure, then a fluid challenge may be given. If this is insufficient to correct the hypotension, a balloon pump should be inserted in the opposite groin. This is good practice whether the case is managed by PCI or surgery. Definitive treatment should then take place.

PERIPROCEDURAL MYOCARDIAL INFARCTION MANAGEMENT

Occasionally the patient will develop pain and ECG changes in the recovery area or on the ward after a procedure. Irrespective of the management plan that has been decided on for the patient – medical therapy, revascularization with PCI or surgical management – the patient should usually be brought back to the lab. If surgery is necessary, a balloon pump should be placed and urgent bypass grafting discussed with surgical colleagues. If PCI or pharmacological management is the preferred option then immediate intervention is often indicated. If there is no intervention on site, but it is indicated, then a balloon pump should be placed, aspirin, clopidogrel and a GP IIb–IIIa inhibitor started and immediate transfer arranged for PCI.

Stroke

Most strokes following cardiac catheterization are embolic in nature. They are reported to have occurred in 0.05 per cent of diagnostic cases in the last SCA&I data set [9] and in 0.001 per cent in a recent UK series [11]. Recent data using transcranial Doppler demonstrates that any manipulation of devices in the aorta will cause the embolization of microparticulate matter, although the majority are fortunately asymptomatic. Not all strokes are atheroembolic (Table 7.7).

The presence of an altered neurological state after angiography is distressing for all concerned. Evaluation by cerebral cross-sectional imaging is necessary to obtain a diagnosis, but this may be delayed. The diagnosis is usually clinically self-evident.

REDUCING THE RISK

Catheter manipulation

All end-hole catheters should be introduced over an appropriate sized, usually 0.035″ guidewire. The guidewire should have an atraumatic J tip to avoid catching the aortic wall and inadvertently lifting atheromatous plaque. Even when a straight wire is needed to cross an aortic valve, the catheter should be taken to the root over a J wire first and then the J wire exchanged for a straight one.

Table 7.7 Causes of stroke directly or indirectly due to cardiac catheterization

	Risk factors
Embolic stroke	Catheter manipulation
	Inadvertent air embolism
	Thrombus injection
	Atheroembolic
Haemorrhagic stroke	Heparin
	Warfarin
	GP IIb–IIIa inhibitors
	Aspirin/clopidogrel

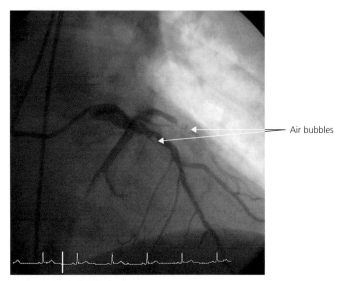

Figure 7.5   Air bubbles in the coronary artery.

Most centres take the J tip wire around into the ascending aorta and deploy the catheter 2–3 cm above the coronary ostium. The catheter is aspirated to ensure there is no air in the system and then connected to a closed system, after ensuring a fluid-to-fluid interface. The catheter is then aspirated again to ensure that no air has been trapped between the catheter tip and the manifold. Some centres use a different practice and deploy the catheter distal to the left subclavian artery, avoiding embolization during the aspiration and flushing procedure. They then take the catheter around the arch. The risk of catching unseen atheromatous plaques in the arch may outweigh the reduction in air embolization.

Careful manifold management

The manifold system should be flushed carefully and maintained air bubble free. When the manifold is flushed and is to be connected to the catheter, it is important to ensure that there is an obvious meniscus of blood at the end of the catheter to allow a fluid–fluid interface. This will avoid unintentionally introducing air into the system. A further safeguard is to then aspirate blood back through the manifold into the contrast syringe prior to the first intracoronary injection and then inject contrast to opacify the catheter in the aortic root, prior to engaging the coronary artery. This avoids injecting air down the coronary artery (Figure 7.5).

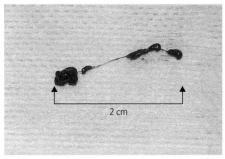

Figure 7.6 Thrombus from catheter equipment.

Wire dwell times

No wire (e.g. a straight wire trying to cross an aortic valve or a J wire trying to cannulate a left subclavian artery for selective left internal mammary artery angiography) should be within a catheter or coronary artery for more than 3 minutes. The wire should be taken out and wiped with heparinized saline and the catheter aspirated. Failure to adhere to short wire dwell times, when the system is not anticoagulated, will increase the risk of a clot developing within the catheter around the wire (Figure 7.6).

Avoid high-risk locations

There are a number of situations where the risk of thrombus is high and the information is either not important or can be obtained in other ways. LV injections are contraindicated when LV thrombus is documented and caution is needed to avoid an apical pigtail catheter position in recent MI. Similarly, in aortic and mitral valve endocarditis, the information from an aortogram and left ventriculogram can be gained by echocardiography.

Cannulation site complications

Cannulation site complications occur in approximately 1 per cent of cases and represent a significant burden of litigation for the cardiologist. Complications may include:

- Haematoma
- False aneurysm

- Arteriovenous fistula
- Retrograde femoral, iliac or aortic dissection
- Concealed bleeding (i.e. retroperitoneal haemotoma)
- Vessel occlusion.

These are discussed in detail in the vascular access sections of Chapters 3 and 4.

Radiation dermatitis

Coronary angiography produces one of the highest radiation exposures of any common X-ray procedure, typically 2–4 Roentgen/minute (R/min) for fluoroscopy and 30–60 R/min for acquisition runs. Doses are particularly high to the patient during angioplasty and electrophysiological procedures, where long periods of fluoroscopic imaging are conducted in limited views. However, when faced with difficult coronary arteries or graft cases, these doses can also occur during diagnostic cases as well. As 1 R of exposure delivers a dose of about 1 rad to soft tissue, the absorbed dose may reach several Gray (1 Gray (Gy) = 100 rad). Exposures of 3–25 Gy are associated with skin manifestations ranging from erythema to necrosis [12,13]. The cumulative dose needed to induce chronic skin changes is thought to be above 10 Gy [14]. There are case reports of radiation dermatitis after prolonged cardiac catheterization [15]. The radiation effects on the skin are listed in Table 7.8.

Erythema may develop immediately or over the first few days. The onset of chronic dermatitis may then develop over a variable interval, ranging from a few weeks to 10 years [15], manifesting as persistent erythema, telangiectasia, fibrosis, atrophy and ulceration and histopathological dermal fibrosis.

The effects of radiation on the skin highlight the need for tight control of radiation exposure to patients and staff. Up-to-date digital

Table 7.8 Radiation effects on skin

Exposure (Gy)	Manifestation
3–10	Erythema
7–10	Permanent epilation
12–25	Moist desquamation
25+	Necrosis

equipment and proper dose monitoring have a crucial role to play. A staff member, usually a radiographer, is always nominated as a radiation safety officer, to ensure that standards of radiation protection are maintained.

Angiography-associated renal dysfunction

Atheroembolic renal dysfunction and contrast nephropathy

A decline in renal function following angiography is usually ascribed to contrast-associated nephropathy. Although this is more common, atheroembolic renal dysfunction can also occur.

ATHEROEMBOLIC RENAL DYSFUNCTION

Atheroembolic renal dysfunction is generally seen in white males over the age of 55 years, and occurs later than contrast nephropathy. Cholesterol emboli from the aortic wall may cause obstructive symptoms and signs as well as provoke an inflammatory response, which may include an allergic component. It tends to develop a week or more after the cardiac catheter and may persist or progress over weeks or months. The overall incidence appears relatively low even in an older patient group (around 2 per cent) [16]. A number of criteria suggest its presence, including:

- Evidence of systemic embolization: livedo reticularis, petechiae, digital infarction or splinter haemorrhage
- Hollenhorst plaques (cholesterol emboli in retinal arteries)
- Eosinophilia: >3 per cent or >350 absolute eosinophil count
- Eosinophiluria: >1 per cent
- Erythrocyte sedimentation rate (ESR) >30 mm/h.

Preventative measures

In older subjects with evidence of peripheral vascular disease evidenced by previous stroke, intermittent claudication or abdominal aortic aneurysm or those who have diabetes or pre-existing renal impairment, minimizing catheter exchanges is probably the only preventative procedure. If catheters need to be changed then changing over a double length exchange 0.035″ guidewire may be required to reduce traumatic abrasion of the aorta, although there is no evidence to support this.

If atheroembolic renal dysfunction does occur, then management is supportive, with renal replacement therapy as required.

CONTRAST NEPHROPATHY

The incidence of contrast nephropathy depends somewhat on the definition applied. These have included a 25 per cent, 50 per cent or even 100 per cent rise in plasma creatinine (P_{Cr}). In a recent epidemiological study in patients undergoing percutaneous intervention, 14.5 per cent showed a 25 per cent rise in P_{Cr}, and 0.8 per cent needed renal replacement therapy. Although the incidence of those subjects needing renal replacement therapy is low, 36 per cent of those who required renal replacement therapy died in hospital and only 20 per cent were alive at the end of two years [17]. The consequences of renal dysfunction in this group are dire.

The administration of contrast causes a decline in renal function in at-risk individuals for a number of reasons. Previously attempts were directed at alleviating the contrast-induced flow changes – initial vasodilatation followed by a more prolonged period of vasoconstriction, using agents such a calcium channel blockers, ACE inhibitors, dopamine and atrial natriuretic peptide (ANP). None showed a benefit. Other concerns were a direct toxic effect renal tubular epithelial cells, precipitation of proteins causing intratubular obstruction and finally free radical damage due to the tenuous nature of intramedullary O_2 tension even in normal healthy kidneys (pO_2 is around 20 mmHg). Little has been done to investigate the direct toxic effects and studies have not confirmed a pressure gradient suggesting intratubular obstruction. The current direction of research is the role of free radicals mediating damage to the ascending loop of Henle.

Those subjects at risk of contrast-induced nephropathy have been well identified as those with:

- Pre-existing renal dysfunction – The rise in P_{Cr} is proportional to the baseline creatinine
- Diabetes
- Intravascular volume depletion

Table 7.9 The relationship between modified Cockcroft formula and serum creatinine

Estimated kidney function (% GFR)	Blood creatinine level (μmol/L)	Renal status
Over 75	60–120	Normal
40–75	110–200	Slightly reduced
15–40	175–350	Markedly reduced
Less than 15	300 upwards	Severe renal dysfunction

GFR, glomerular filtration rate.

- High volumes of contrast – The rise in P_{Cr} is proportional to the volume of contrast. No contrast nephropathy has been reported with volumes less than 100 mL of contrast
- High osmolar contrast media
- Concomitant nephrotoxic medication (e.g. NSAIDs).

Increasing age and the coexistence of heart failure are also cited, but this may reflect the overestimation of renal function in the elderly, where a normal P_{Cr} level may reflect low muscle mass, rather than normal renal function. The estimation of creatinine clearance utilizing the modified Cockcroft–Gault formula is a better way of assessing the likely risk of contrast-induced nephropathy in those subjects with low glomerular filtration rates (Table 7.9). Heart failure subjects are often mildly volume depleted because of the co-prescription of diuretics.

In contrast to atheroembolic renal failure, contrast nephropathy occurs between two and seven days after the angiographic procedure, with the peak rise in P_{Cr} occurring on day 4–5. An estimation of P_{Cr} at 72 hours will identify 90 per cent of affected subjects. In UK practice, this will involve collaboration between the cardiology service and the general practitioner.

Preventive measures
There have been a number of trials investigating strategies to prevent contrast nephropathy. These have included dopamine, calcium channel blockers, ANP, ACE inhibitors, theophylline and endothelin antagonists. The only effective strategy has been prehydration with 0.45 per cent saline, although there is probably not much difference between 0.45 per cent and 0.9 per cent saline in practice. Some interesting data have been seen with pretreatment with oral N-acetylcysteine with low volumes of contrast in CT scanning in patients with renal dysfunction, but whether

this is maintained in procedures with higher contrast volumes is currently under investigation. We currently use oral N-acetylcysteine, but recognize that the evidence supporting this strategy is debated. The management of at-risk renal patients is as follows:

Urgent cases

1. *Identify those at risk*: Diabetes, impaired renal function and volume depletion. Stop unnecessary nephrotoxic agents (NSAIDs, diuretics if possible) and if indicated, proceed to catheter-based investigation.
2. *Pre procedure*: Intravenous infusion of 250 mL of 0.9 per cent saline per 0.5 hour up to 500 mL. This has to be tempered by clinical assessment of cardiac function. Oral N-acetylcysteine 600 mg twice daily for 48 hours.
3. *Post procedure*: Intravenous infusion of 1 L of 0.9 per cent saline over 12 hours. Assessment of P_{Cr} at 12 hours and 72 hours. Oral N-acetylcysteine 600 mg twice daily for 48 hours.

Non-urgent cases

1. *Identify those at risk*: Presence of diabetes, elevated plasma creatinine or volume depletion.
2. *Stop nephrotoxic agents*: Non-steroidal anti-inflammatory drugs (NSAIDs), diuretics if possible.
3. *Pre hydrate*: 1 L 0.9 per cent saline for 12 hours pre catheterization.
4. *Post hydrate*: 1 L 0.9 per cent saline for 12 hours post catheterization.
5. *Postcatheter care*: Assessment of P_{Cr} at 12 hours and 72 hours. The second assessment of creatinine may need to be done by the patient's general practitioner.

Management of deranged renal function

There is no magic bullet for the management of worsening renal function. The prompt involvement of a renal physician and the early use of renal replacement therapy may be necessary to allow renal function to recover, and does not necessarily suggest a permanent decline in renal function is likely. Unfortunately, recognition and preventative treatment or timely postprocedural management does not always mean that a recovery is possible either.

References

1. Goss JE, Chambers CE, Heupler FA, Jr. Systemic anaphylactoid reactions to iodinated contrast media during cardiac catheterization

procedures: guidelines for prevention, diagnosis, and treatment. Laboratory Performance Standards Committee of the Society for Cardiac Angiography and Interventions. *Cathet Cardiovasc Diag* 1995; **34:** 99–104.

2. Thomsen HS, Bush WH. Treatment of the adverse effects of contrast media. *Acta Radiol* 1998; **39:** 212–218.

3. Siegle RL, Halvorsen RA, Dillon J *et al.* The use of iohexol in patients with previous reactions to ionic contrast material. A multicenter clinical trial. *Investig Radiol* 1991; **26:** 411–416.

4. Enright T, Chua-Lim A, Duda E *et al.* The role of a documented allergic profile as a risk factor for radiographic contrast media reaction. *Ann Allergy* 1989; **62:** 302–305.

5. Lang DM, Alpern MB, Visintainer PF *et al.* Increased risk for anaphylactoid reaction from contrast media in patients on beta-adrenergic blockers or with asthma. *Ann Intern Med* 1991; **115:** 270–276.

6. Ritchie JL, Nissen SE, Douglas JSJ *et al.* Use of nonionic or low osmolar contrast agents in cardiovascular procedures. American College of Cardiology Cardiovascular Imaging Committee. *J Am Coll Cardiol* 1993; **21:** 269–273.

7. Epstein AE, Hallstrom AP, Rogers WJ *et al.* Mortality following ventricular arrhythmia suppression by encainide, flecainide, and moricizine after myocardial infarction. The original design concept of the Cardiac Arrhythmia Suppression Trial (CAST). *JAMA* 1993; **270:** 2451–2455.

8. Sprung CL, Pozen RG, Rozanski JJ *et al.* Advanced ventricular arrhythmias during bedside pulmonary artery catheterization. *Am J Med* 1982; **72:** 203–208.

9. Noto TJJ, Johnson LW, Krone R *et al.* Cardiac catheterization 1990: a report of the Registry of the Society for Cardiac Angiography and Interventions (SCA&I). *Cathet Cardiovasc Diag* 1991; **24:** 75–83.

10. Tsang TS, Freeman WK, Barnes ME *et al.* Rescue echocardiographically guided pericardiocentesis for cardiac perforation complicating catheter-based procedures. The Mayo Clinic experience. *J Am Coll Cardiol* 1998; **32:** 1345–1350.

11. Papaconstantinou HDF, Marshall AJF, Burrell CJ. Diagnostic cardiac catheterization in a hospital without on-site cardiac surgery. *Heart* 1999; **81:** 465–469.

12. Nahass GT. Acute radiodermatitis after radiofrequency catheter ablation. *J Am Acad Dermatol* 1997; **36:** 881–884.

13. Nenot JC. Medical and surgical management for localized radiation injuries. *Int J Radiat Biol* 1990; **57:** 783–795.
14. Balter S. Guidelines for personnel radiation monitoring in the cardiac catheterization laboratory. Laboratory Performance Standards Committee of the Society for Cardiac Angiography and Interventions. *Cathet Cardiovasc Diag* 1993; **30:** 277–279.
15. Dehen L, Vilmer C, Humiliere C *et al.* Chronic radiodermatitis following cardiac catheterization: a report of two cases and a brief review of the literature. *Heart* 1999; **81:** 308–312.
16. Saklayen MG, Gupta S, Suryaprasad A *et al.* Incidence of atheroembolic renal failure after coronary angiography. A prospective study. *Angiology* 1997; **48:** 609–613.
17. McCullough PA, Wolyn R, Rocher LL *et al.* Acute renal failure after coronary intervention: incidence, risk factors, and relationship to mortality. *Am J Med* 1997; **103:** 368–375.

Emergency procedures

8

Intra-aortic balloon pump

The intra-aortic balloon pump is a crucial adjunctive treatment for cardiogenic shock and preshock and blood flow augmentation in critical left main stem disease and/or medically refractory angina. All angiographic centres should have the capability to insert a balloon pump in an emergency. This can stabilize a patient until a definitive procedure is available, even if that necessitates transfer. Balloon pumps should be seen as a bridge to a definitive treatment and not as a treatment *per se.*

Background

The intra-aortic balloon pump (IABP) is a polyurethane balloon capable of rapid inflation and deflation by means of an external pump. Expansion of the balloon in diastole increases aortic volume and pressure. This increases the pressure in the aorta, including the aortic root, increasing the perfusion pressure gradient across coronary arteries which should in turn increase flow. The rapid collapse in systole reduces afterload by reducing volume and therefore pressure in the aorta. This has the effect of decreasing afterload, cardiac work, myocardial oxygen

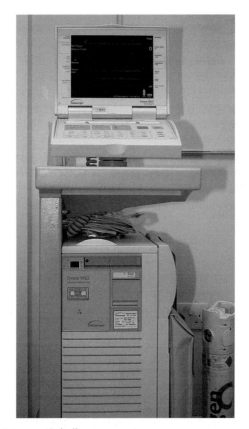

Figure 8.1   Intra-aortic balloon pump.

requirements and increasing cardiac output. The increased left ventricular (LV) emptying improves forward flow and decreases left heart filling pressures, but relies on a competent aortic valve to work (Figures 8.1 and 8.2).

Cardiogenic shock

Balloon pumping in cardiogenic shock is associated with a reduction in wall stress, and increase in coronary flow and a concomitant reduction in ischaemia. There is usually an increase in mean arterial pressure, and cardiac index and LV filling pressure fall significantly. There is usually a

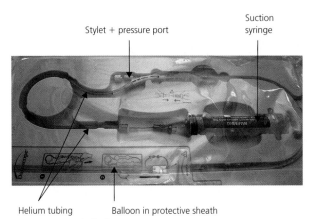

Figure 8.2   Intra-aortic balloon.

marked rise in diastolic pressure, but the effect on cardiac output is not easy to predict. The beneficial effect of balloon pumping may only improve coronary flow when the pressure falls below the threshold at which autoregulation can maintain flow (40–60 mmHg). In profound shock, however, both coronary flow and cardiac output commonly increase.

Cardiogenic shock has a very poor outcome with a one-year mortality between 50 per cent and 80 per cent. The earlier the downward spiral to cardiovascular collapse is interrupted, the easier it may be to reverse and the better the results. An IABP is beneficial if there is an associated mechanical defect such as a ventricular septal defect (VSD) or acute severe mitral regurgitation (MR). It is less effective in primary pump failure.

The importance of IABP as a bridging procedure to a definitive treatment is shown by data from the SHOCK Registry, where early revascularization (<24 hours) was associated with a 77 per cent survival rate compared with only 10 per cent in those who had delayed revascularization (>24 hours) [1].

Cardiogenic shock due to acute myocarditis may be different, as there is a degree of recoverability. Some data suggest that IABP was of benefit even in those in whom pharmacological support had failed. Longer term circulatory support with ventricular assist devices allowed full recovery in most patients [2].

Refractory ischaemia

Refractory ischaemia provides the single largest indication for IABP insertion. In the presence of normal blood pressure, the haemodynamic effects are often small with only small changes in cardiac output and filling pressures. In particular, there may be little increase in flow across a critical coronary stenosis [3] unless in the presence of shock, where there may be a rapid increase in flow. Following myocardial infarction (MI), the Thrombolysis and Angioplasty in Myocardial Infarction (TAMI) study demonstrated a reduced reocclusion rate [4]. Other data suggest that in patients with failed angioplasty, IABP for 48 hours improved vessel patency.

Bridge to revascularization or transplantation

Patients who have an unsuccessful percutaneous intervention (PCI) that requires urgent bypass grafting are unusual in current practice. However, if they are hypotensive or having ongoing pain due to reduced coronary flow, then the insertion of an IABP may be indicated.

Patients with shock or preshock, who are transplantation candidates, occasionally need assisted circulatory support, although the necessary duration of support usually requires percutaneous cardiopulmonary support (or extracorporeal membranous oxygenation) or the implantation of a ventricular assist device, where these options are available. IABP can provide short-term support until a more long-term circulatory supportive strategy can be arranged. Practically, in the UK, this is a rare use of IABP support.

Indications and contraindications

The indications and contraindications for IABP are listed in Table 8.1.

Insertion and management of balloon pumps

Modern aortic balloons are compatible with 8F sheaths and vary between 25 and 50 mL. Most UK centres insert two sizes: 34 mL for small adults (<163 cm) and 40 mL (>163 cm) for all others. Each individual manufacturer gives size ranges for each balloon depending on the patient's height. Datascope, for example, suggest 25 cc (25 mL) for patients <5'0" (<152 cm), 34 cc (34 mL) for 5'0"–5'4" (152–163 cm),

Table 8.1 Indications and contraindications for intra-aortic balloon pump insertion

Indications	Haemodynamic compromise
	Cardiogenic shock (MI, VSD, mitral regurgitation or failed PCI)
	Failure to wean from bypass
	Pretransplantation support
	Medical refractory ischaemia
	Unstable angina pre PCI/CABG
	Prophylactic support
	High risk PCI
	Stabilization with severe aortic stenosis
	Critical coronary disease without rest pain pre PCI/CABG
Contraindications	Moderate/severe aortic regurgitation
	Abdominal or low thoracic aortic aneurysm
	Aortic dissection
	Sepsis
	Uncontrolled bleeding diathesis
	Severe peripheral vascular disease

MI, myocardial infarction; VSD, ventricular septal defect; PCI, percutaneous intervention; CABG, coronary artery bypass graft.

40 cc (40 mL) for 5′4″–6′0″ (163–183 cm) and 50 cc (50 mL) for >6′0″ (>183 cm) for their kit. Particular expertise in the setting up and subsequent physiological management of balloon pumps is usually the province of perfusionists or physiology technicians.

An IABP following an angiogram or angioplasty for preshock or cardiogenic shock is usually inserted through the existing vascular access site after performing a sheath exchange for the 8F IABP sheath. It is possible to insert a 34 mL or 40 mL IABP without a sheath through a 6F sheath site, but sheath sizes larger than this usually have a degree of blood leakage around the puncture site and an 8F sheath would need to be inserted to control this. An IABP inserted preprocedurally is normally placed in the contralateral femoral artery.

INSERTION TECHNIQUE

The balloon is prepared according to the manufacturer's instruction. This will involve the following steps, although only the steps concerning the physician will be discussed below:

- Setting up of pump
- Setting up pressure bags and connectors
- Obtaining arterial access
- Preparing the balloon
- Inserting the balloon
- Connecting the balloon to pump
- Initiating pumping.

Arterial access

The technique of femoral artery cannulation is described in chapter 4, as part of femoral vascular access. Once needle access is gained, the long floppy IABP wire is taken and placed in the ascending aorta, around the aortic arch. The puncture site is predilated with the accompanying dilator and then the 8F sheath is inserted as previously discussed. The wire is left in place. If the balloon is to be inserted sheathless, the balloon is inserted next. In some balloon pump kits the sheath has to be assembled first and careful attention should be paid to removal of the dilator without damaging the haemostatic valve. There may be some small leakage of blood through the haemostatic valve which settles with balloon insertion.

Preparing the balloon

Once arterial access has been achieved, the balloon is opened and prepared. Initially, the plastic tubing that connects the balloon and pump is taken and the one-way valve connected, leaving the bulk of the balloon in the tray for ease of handling. A 60 mL syringe is connected and negative pressure applied to aspirate 30 mL of volume from the balloon. The syringe and one-way valve are then removed, followed by the stylet from the central balloon lumen. The guidewire is wiped with a damp swab and then backloaded through the central lumen of the balloon. The balloon is threaded along the wire until the guidewire passes out of the distal end of the balloon. The balloon is then passed through the haemostatic valve and advanced. There should be no resistance to passing the balloon. Any resistance usually indicates aorto-iliac disease. The balloon should be withdrawn and the aorto-iliac segment reassessed by angiography.

The balloon is advanced to a position 2 cm distal to the origin of the left subclavian artery, which is level with the tracheal bifurcation. This should always be confirmed with either plane film X-ray if it was not screened in with ciné, or a stored angiographic frame. The sheath should then be pulled back 2–3 cm to ensure that the whole balloon is out of the sheath.

Next the guidewire is removed and 3 mL of blood aspirated and the balloon flushed first with a hand injection of saline and then for 10 seconds via the pressure transducer tubing. Finally the helium tubing is passed to the technician and connected to the pump.

The sheath and balloon are both fixed with two non-absorbable sutures. Then the sheath seal is passed down the catheter to the introducer hub and the seal connected to the hub. Occasionally you come across a situation in which a sheath has been stitched in, but the balloon has not been fixed at all, which leaves it at risk of being pulled distally, increasing the risk of barotraumas to the iliac artery.

Pitfalls

- *Bleeding*: Blood can appear to be leaking at several points in the insertion procedure when least expected. The first is when the 8F dilator is removed from the 8F sheath. Blood can leak back at this time and this can be stopped by pinching the sheath below the haemostatic valve if the bleeding is marked or allow it to settle when the balloon is inserted. The next source of blood is when the balloon is being inserted into the sheath and blood starts to appear through the upper folds of the balloon. This is caused by blood tracking up the folds of the balloon and will disappear when the balloon is entirely intraluminal. The last point of unwanted bleeding is when the sheath seal is connected to the introducer sheath hub. If this happens then a suture can be passed around the seal to secure haemostasis.
- Never take blood samples through the pressure monitoring line.
- If the pressure monitoring trace becomes damped, aspirate and flush for 15 seconds. If it clears, leave connected. If blood cannot be aspirated easily or the pressure trace remains damped off, then it must be assumed to have thrombus within the lumen and should be capped off permanently.
- Always maintain heparinized flush at 300 mmHg to ensure central lumen patency.

Starting pumping

Once all is connected, the technician will initiate pumping after priming and setting the balloon pump console. Normally this is at 2:1 to set timing of inflation and deflation and to check balloon integrity. Once all is working correctly, the 1:1 augmentation is started.

Removing the balloon pump

The pressure line and gas connections are disconnected. The balloon will collapse with aortic pressure and there is no need to aspirate the balloon. Cut the fixing sutures first. Then grip the introducer sheath with your left hand and pull the balloon back to the sheath, but do not pull it into the sheath. Then with a smooth movement pull the sheath and the balloon out together as one unit. If there is excessive resistance, it may need to be removed by arteriotomy. Allow 3–4 spurts of blood from the puncture site to clear clot and then apply digital pressure over the arterial puncture site, remembering that this is 2–3 cm above the skin puncture site. Usually 20–30 minutes is necessary, partly because of the duration the sheath has been *in situ*, which markedly reduces femoral arterial elastic recoil, and partly because of the calibre of the puncture in the femoral artery.

Sheathless insertion

Many operators introduce IABPs without a sheath. The only difference is that after wire access is gained, the puncture is not dilated until the balloon is ready to be inserted. Care should be taken to insert the balloon without kinking it. This can be reduced with adequate predilatation and with some countertraction on the wire at the point of insertion. If the IABP is being inserted after a diagnostic/therapeutic procedure and a sheath is already been in place, then we would not insert the balloon sheathless unless the sheath was 6F or less, as problems can occur with haemostasis. On removal, the balloon can be pulled straight out.

The advantages of sheathless insertion are clear in smaller subjects who are more likely to suffer from occlusive flow problems in the femoral artery, and in those with peripheral arterial disease.

Maximizing augmentation

The essence of balloon pump technology is the timing of the balloon expansion and deflation. The balloon can be triggered by various mechanisms such as the R wave, a pacing spike, systolic pressure trace and at a fixed rate. Most cases are triggered by the R wave (Table 8.2).

Table 8.2 Mechanisms of intra-aortic balloon pump triggering

Trigger	Indication
R wave	Normal mode
Pacing spike	VVI/DDD pacing
Systolic pressure	Difficulty with R wave tracking or pacing or the presence of atrial fibrillation
Fixed rate	Asystole or cardiac arrest

Setting the timings of the balloon pump is normally done by the perfusionists or physiology technicians. However all physicians who insert IABPs should be able to set them up. Fortunately most are self-adjusting. Ideally, fine-tuning the timing of balloon inflation and deflation should be done when the pump is set 2:1. The inflation and deflation can be too early or too late.

If possible, balloon inflation should occur promptly at the onset of diastole, which coincides with the diacrotic notch on the aortic pressure trace. On inflation, there should be a sharp 'V' on the pressure waveform. Deflation should occur just prior to systole, resulting in a reduction in aortic end-diastolic and systolic pressure (Figure 8.3).

- *Early inflation*: If the onset of balloon inflation is before the dicrotic notch it leads to a blurring of the pressure trace from unassisted systole and assisted diastole. Potentially this can prematurely close the aortic valve, increase left ventricular end-diastolic pressure, increase afterload, provoke aortic regurgitation and increase myocardial oxygen demand.
- *Late inflation*: If the onset of balloon inflation occurs after the dicrotic notch, the 'V' pre-balloon inflation is not sharp. This results in suboptimal coronary perfusion because the augmented pressure is less.
- *Early deflation*: In this situation the inflation is well timed with a sharp 'V' and good initial augmentation, but the pressure falls off early, resulting in suboptimal coronary perfusion. The assisted end-diastolic pressure may be lower than expected and the assisted systolic pressure higher than expected. Overall this has the potential to reverse blood flow in the coronary arteries, providing less effective afterload reduction and increased myocardial oxygen demand (Figure 8.4, page 257).

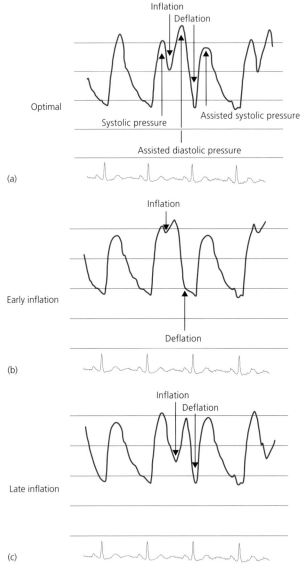

Figure 8.3 Intra-aortic balloon pump pressure traces: normal and suboptimal inflation traces.

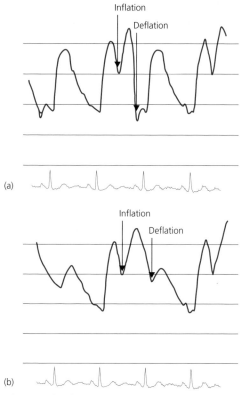

Figure 8.4 Suboptimal deflation timing. (a) Early deflation; (b) late deflation.

- *Late deflation*: The balloon inflates normally with a good 'V' and there is good augmentation. The balloon deflates late, increasing aortic pressure in early systole, which prevents any afterload reduction and may increase afterload and increase oxygen demand.

Ongoing management

ANTICOAGULATION

Most centres anticoagulate patients with a balloon pump *in situ*. The activated partial thromboplastin time (APPT) should be between two and three times normal using intravenous unfractionated heparin.

Table 8.3 Daily checks for an intra-aortic balloon pump

Distal pulses (every nursing shift)	A decline in recorded foot pulse or an ankle brachial index (the ratio of Doppler systolic pressure in the foot/ Doppler pressure in the upper arm) <0.5 indicates serious ischaemia
Platelet count	Usually falls with balloon pumping to between 50 and 100 × 10^3/mL, but recovers after pumping stops. Further falls may represent HITS (heparin-induced thrombocytopenia) or clumping if abciximab has been administered
Temperature	

DAILY CHECKS

The checks listed in Table 8.3 should be carried out every day.

Complications

Possible complications of IABP include the following:

- Limb ischaemia (pre-existing arterial disease, atheroembolic disease, arterial dissection)
- Cerebrovascular accident (CVA)
- Sepsis
- Balloon rupture
- Thrombocytopenia
- Bleeding.

LIMB ISCHAEMIA

Ischaemia can be due to pre-existing vascular disease, thrombus, dissection or there may be embolization of atheromatous material. Ischaemia is particularly common in people with pre-existing aorto-ilio-femoral vascular disease. It is much more common with older, larger calibre IABP, but even 8F systems can cause vascular insufficiency. Presentation may be soon after balloon insertion. If severe ipsilateral ischaemia develops, then causes may include inserting the balloon distal to the common femoral artery, the presence of severe local vascular disease or a vascular complication higher up at the level of aortic bifurcation and proximal iliac artery. The balloon pump should be removed and an attempt made to place it in the contralateral leg. The overall risk of severe limb ischaemia needing removal of the pump is approximately 5 per cent [5]. The ultimate risk is that the limb may not be salvageable.

Arterial dissection can occur in the aorta, iliac or femoral arteries. It can either be caused at the time of balloon insertion or as a result of the process of balloon inflation/deflation. Caution is necessary at the time of insertion if the wire or balloon will not advance. If there is difficulty, one strategy is to place a small 4F sheath or 5F dilator and confirm that you are in the true lumen. If there is significant aorto-iliac disease then the balloon should not be inserted. Occasionally it is necessary to place an IABP even in the presence of suboptimal anatomy if the consequences of not doing so are high. In this situation it is better to confirm you are in true lumen and then place the wire in the aortic arch through a steerable, small-calibre diagnostic catheter such as a Judkins right 4 (JR4).

Atheromatous material can embolize from the aortic wall, which may cause limb ichaemia. Evidence of systemic embolization includes livedo reticularis, petechiae, digital infarction or splinter haemorrage, an eosinophilia (>3 per cent or >350 absolute eosinophil count), eosinophiluria (>1 per cent) or a raised ESR (>30 mm/h).

CEREBROVASCULAR ACCIDENT

CVA is a rare complication and only occurs if the there is balloon rupture, the balloon is placed too high in the aorta or there is extensive dissection.

SEPSIS

Meticulous nursing and medical care is important. There is some evidence that sepsis is not important until the pump has been in for seven days or more. However, a confirmed bacteraemia is a definite indication to remove the balloon.

BALLOON RUPTURE

This is also rare and indicates either mistreatment of the balloon on insertion or the presence of calcific vascular disease which erodes through the balloon. It can vary from a very small leak to catastrophic rupture. Advances in manufacture mean this is now very uncommon.

Helium is almost insoluble in blood and the resulting air embolism is very difficult to treat, often requiring prolonged episodes of hyperbaric oxygen therapy to maintain tissue viability until the helium has dispersed. The balloon pump usually picks up small leaks with its own autodiagnostic algorithms, but occasionally the first finding is blood in the extracorporeal tubing or a sudden change in the diastolic waveform.

The immediate priority is to stop pumping and to remove the balloon. Failure to act promptly can allow blood to clot within the balloon, which may then need surgical removal.

THROMBOCYTOPENIA

The platelet count normally falls with balloon pumping to between 50 and 100×10^3/ml, but recovers after pumping stops. If the platelet count is lower than this, or does not rise after the cessation of IABP support, then another cause such as heparin-induced thrombocytopenia should be considered. Other causes of thrombocytopenia may include the administration of abciximab (ReoPro) at the time of catheter intervention or a pre-existing platelet abnormality.

BLEEDING

Bleeding can occur at the vascular access site and may be due to excessive anticoagulation, sheath movement (in an agitated patient) or local arterial trauma. This can be managed with local pressure, occasionally using a FemoStop compression device, as long as distal flow is preserved. If this does not stop bleeding, a local surgical repair may be needed.

Temporary transvenous pacing

The insertion of a temporary pacing wire is a key skill for the cardiologist. There are two major groups of patients who require temporary pacing: those with classical indications for antibradycardia pacing and those who require pacing-delivered antitachycardia treatment.

Patients requiring pacing for bradycardia include those in whom a pacing wire is inserted proactively for procedures likely to cause bradycardia, such as rotational atherectomy. It also includes those for whom an existing bradycardia needs to be treated to improve haemodynamic stability, for example in the context of an inferior MI complicated by complete heart block, where the loss of AV synchrony and bradycardia causes haemodynamic compromise. Finally, a bradycardia induced within the lab which pharmacological strategies have failed to correct may be dramatically improved by pacing strategies; an example would be a profound vagal reaction associated with bradycardia.

Pacing may also be very useful to treat and/or suppress brady-arrhythmia during procedures in acutely unwell patients.

Indications for temporary pacing

ATRIOVENTRICULAR BLOCK (FIGURE 8.5)

First-degree atrioventricular (AV) block does not require pacing. Second-degree AV block may be either Mobitz type I or type II:

- *Mobitz type I (Wenckebach)*: This is the incremental increase in PR interval as the AV nodal conduction slows, until the P wave is not conducted. The PR are interval is then reset and the process begins again. It is primarily due to AV node dysfunction. It does not need pacing unless there is a degree of associated bradycardia with haemodynamic compromise. The threshold for pacing is lower if it

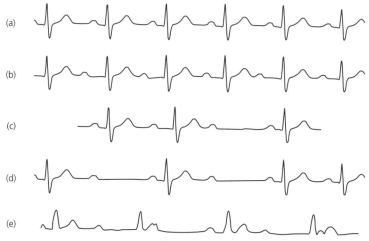

Figure 8.5 Atrioventricular nodal block. (a) Normal; (b) first-degree block; (c) second-degree block 'Wenckebach' or Mobitz type I; (d) second-degree block or Mobitz type II; (e) third-degree block or complete heart block.

is in the context of an anterior MI, which indicates a larger area of ischaemia, or the patient is likely to undergo PCI.

• *Mobitz type II*: This is where the PR interval is fixed, but some P waves may be blocked so that some are conducted and some are not. It may be in a regular pattern such as 2:1 or 3:1 block. It is less stable than type I block, usually because of associated distal fascicular block and usually warrants pacing if the rate is slow, or associated with haemodynamic instability or an anterior MI. Similarly, if there is the likelihood of PCI, a prophylactically placed pacing wire may be advantageous.

Third-degree AV block, or complete heart block, is where there is complete AV dissociation. The P waves occur independently of the QRS complexes. If it has occurred because of gradual AV node disease and troponin or CK-MB assay is normal and the patient is haemodynami-cally stable this does not require temporarily pacing. The patient can wait until a permanent system is implanted. Haemodynamic stability is usually associated with a faster ventricular rate (>50 bpm) and narrow QRS complexes (<0.12 ms).

In the context of myocardial infarction, permanent pacing is not normally undertaken for one week post MI, to see if the AV node can recover. If at 5–7 days there is still evidence of second- or third-degree AV block, then the patient warrants permanent pacing. Any associated haemodynamic instability warrants the insertion of a pacing wire. The occurrence of complete heart block complicating an anterior MI or the likelihood of PCI suggests a lower threshold for pacing should be used.

BUNDLE BRANCH BLOCK

This does not need pacing unless associated with a bradycardia causing haemodynamic compromise.

SINUS BRADYCARDIA

Most sinus bradycardia and sinus arrest is well tolerated and does not require pacing. If there is associated haemodynamic compromise then a pacing wire should be inserted.

CATHETER LAB

In the catheter lab, most arrhythmias that require pacing are managed from the ipsilateral femoral vein to the arterial puncture, because it is often already sterile, draped and readily accessible. The ready access outweighs the small (but definite) increase in risk of an AV fistula and issues regarding sterility.

Most sinus bradycardia is due to high vagal tone, most commonly at the time of sheath insertion and removal or during episodes of pain. It normally passes without incident, but if more profound or associated with hypotension, then atropine should be given (0.6 mg i.v.). If this fails to reverse it, then a pacing wire should be inserted. Previously, beta-agonists such as isoprenaline were used. However, it is often quicker to insert a pacing wire, and probably less proarrhythmogenic.

Similarly with second and third-degree AV block, high vagal tone should be suspected and the first step should be the administration of atropine, although it may be less useful. If resolution does not occur with up to 1.2 mg of atropine, then a pacing wire should be inserted.

Technique

Venous access is discussed in Chapters 3 and 4. It is important to avoid upper body access sites on the non-dominant side, which will make permanent pacing access more difficult.

Once venous access is obtained, the pacing wire and connectors are taken onto the trolley and checked to ensure compatibility. The pacing wire is introduced and advanced to the right atrium (RA). The pacing wire has a fixed curve, to enable steering and is relatively stiff and there are higher risks associated with its manipulation, especially when temporary pacing is taking place in the context of an inferior MI. The pacing wire can catch any of the inferior vena cava (IVC) branches on the way up to the RA, and it should be screened up with fluoroscopy.

ADVANCING THE WIRE INTO THE RIGHT VENTRICLE

If the pacing wire has been inserted from the femoral vein, then the natural curve of the pacing wire may take it across the tricuspid valve (TV). If this fails, there are a number of techniques for crossing the TV. The first involves catching the tip if the pacing wire on the lateral aspect (free wall) of the RA and forming a loop, which prolapses into the right ventricle (RV). It is also possible to catch the intra-atrial septum to the same effect. Withdrawal associated with clockwise torque on the pacing wire causes the tip to flick into the RV. The wire is then advanced into

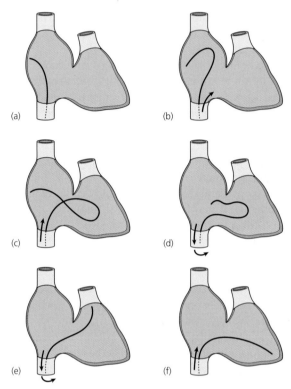

Figure 8.6   Technique 1 for temporary pacing wire insertion.

the RV apex for stable temporary pacing. The wire often needs to be rotated after entering the RV, as it tends to point upwards toward 1–3 o'clock, and ideally should end up pointing towards 4–5 o'clock. This technique has the advantage that the pacing wire tip rarely enters the cardiac veins (Figure 8.6).

Alternatively, instead of the tip catching on the medial aspect of the RA, it can be deflected towards the TV and then once across, a little retraction on the catheter to remove the extra loop in the atrium followed by advancement with counterclockwise twist will deflect the tip of the wire up and down to the apex (Figure 8.7).

The alternative is to try and cross the valve directly. This is easier via the femoral approach. The pacing wire is positioned so that the

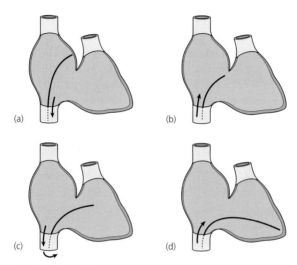

Figure 8.7 Technique 2 for temporary pacing wire insertion.

tip points to 9–10 o'clock and then is rotated clockwise, to point at 2–3 o'clock, at the same time advancing the wire. It should cross the valve, if it does not, withdraw and try again. Common problems are entry into the coronary sinus. This can be seen by changing the camera angle to left anterior oblique (LAO) or right anterior oblique (RAO) 30°. Engaging the coronary sinus in RAO 30° will carry the catheter posteriorly, whereas entering the RV will be anteriorly located. In LAO, the pacing wire will appear to be coming at you in the coronary sinus.

Passage into the RV cavity is normally accompanied by ventricular ectopy, and occasionally by ventricular tachycardia (VT), ventricular fibrillation (VF) or ventricular standstill. If the approach has been from the superior vena cava, then often clockwise torque is required to direct the catheter towards the apex, counterclockwise if an inferior caval approach has been chosen. Once a good position in the RV has been achieved, the pacing wire is connected up. A good position is suggested by a lead position pointing to 4–5 o'clock and almost to the edge of the cardiac silhouette. An endocardial electrogram should show an injury current morphology and it should pace with a left bundle branch block (LBBB) morphology. Right bundle branch block (RBBB) suggests either perforation, coronary sinus or LV pacing.

The threshold should be checked, and should be less than 1.0 V at 1.0 ms pulse width. A higher threshold suggests a suboptimal location or the presence of RV scarring. The pacing wire should be repositioned. The pacing rate is normally set at 70 bpm, with a voltage set at the threshold $+2$ V (e.g. a threshold of 0.4 V suggests pacing at 2.4 V for an adequate margin of safety). A higher rate may be required in other circumstances, such as ectopic suppression for VT prophylaxis.

TEMPORARY ATRIOVENTRICULAR SEQUENTIAL PACING

The only indication for AV sequential pacing is the occurrence of shock or preshock with pure right-side MI and complete heart block. Few centres are equipped with dual temporary pacing boxes unless they are cardiothoracic surgical units.

Two methods are available: the use of preshaped atrial temporary wires and the use of a standard temporary pacing wire. Preshaped leads are only suitable for atrial pacing from the superior vena caval approach and standard leads are only suitable for pacing from the femoral approach. The aim is to place the tip in the atrial appendage, although occasionally atrial pacing can be achieved from the coronary sinus. It should only be attempted by those used to placing permanent atrial leads.

SECURING THE PACING WIRE

In the catheter lab, sheaths are not normally fixed in place during the procedure and neither are the catheters. It may be prudent to place a pacing wire and connector underneath a sterile drape and continue the procedure on top of this to avoid snagging the pacing wire during catheter manipulation. If the pacing wire has been placed for another reason and the pacing wire is going to be left in place, then both the sheath *and* the pacing wire should be fixed. Choose non-absorbable sutures and fix the sheath to the skin and then separately fix the pacing wire to the sheath.

Complications

FAILURE TO PACE/SENSE

Failure to pace/sense in a patient with a pacing wire *in situ* is usually due to migration of the tip. The wire should be repositioned. It is always worth checking the connections and the workings of the pacing box.

PERFORATION

This is suggested by a loss of pacing, with or without signs of pericardial irritation. It is surprisingly common, and reported in up to 30 per cent of cases and is underrecognized clinically. Pericarditis occurs in 5 per cent of perforations and tamponade in 1 per cent [6] (Table 8.4).

The diagnosis can be made by checking the endocardial electrogram, which will demonstrate a morphology change from LBBB to RBBB. The wire needs repositioning, which can normally be done safely, as there is not usually a problem with ongoing bleeding into the pericardial cavity.

PNEUMOTHORAX

A small pneumothorax (<10 per cent) can be left alone, but should be re X-rayed 24 hours later to ensure no progression. A mild to moderate pneumothorax (10–25 per cent) can be aspirated by needle and syringe from the anterior chest wall. A moderate to large pneumothorax will need a chest drain to be placed.

INFECTION

Normally, antibiotic prophylaxis is not required for pacing wire insertion. However, as with all indwelling lines, meticulous attention to asepsis is necessary as a reported incidence of infection is 3–5 per cent [6]. The femoral site is more likely to develop infection than other sites of venous access. The presence of a spiking temperature or a bacteraemia is an indication for removal and culturing of the pacing wire.

Table 8.4 Symptoms and sign of ventricular perforation in temporary transvenous pacing

Symptoms	Chest pain – pericarditic
	Shoulder tip pain
	Shortness of breath (if tamponade present)
Signs	Sudden change in pacing morphology LBBB to RBBB
	Sudden change in threshold
	Loss of pace/sensing
	Pericardial rub
	Pulsus paradoxus (if tamponade present)

HAEMORRHAGE

This can occur from any venous access route, but the major concern is from the subclavian route, where the subclavian artery may be inadvertently punctured. Because of the anatomy, the subclavian artery cannot be compressed externally and may continue to bleed. It may present with chest pain or a new pleural effusion. A new effusion should be tapped to exclude a haemothorax if there has been a recent subclavian puncture.

ARRHYTHMIAS

The insertion of a pacing wire can provoke atrial ectopy in the RA, VT and even VF in the RV. VT can also be stimulated purely by the wire being present. A guide to this is that the VT has a similar morphology to the paced rhythm.

THROMBOEMBOLIC EVENTS

Femoral lines are the only ones studied. A third of pacing wires were associated with thrombus, of which 60 per cent had evidence of pulmonary embolism [6].

Pericardiocentesis

Cardiac tamponade can occur quickly and with dire consequences. However it can also occur more slowly after a catheterization, and may not manifest itself for an hour or two. The ability to recognize and deal with tamponade quickly is very important to the catheter lab doctor.

Broadly there are two groups of patients who require pericardiocentesis: those who come to the catheter lab for drainage of a pre-existing effusion and those in whom the effusion is a complication of the procedure. The technique of drainage is the same.

Background

The onset of tamponade is due to a balance of the rate of fluid accumulation, the distensibility of the pericardium and the intracardiac pressure. There is normally less than 50 mL of fluid in the pericardial space. If 150 mL of fluid accumulates rapidly, then intrapericardial pressure will rise and equal intra-atrial pressure, which then causes right atrial diastolic collapse on echocardiography. If a further increase in fluid volume occurs then eventually the intrapericardial pressure will reach systolic levels and systolic collapse may occur.

The physiological response to tamponade is initially a reflex sympathetically mediated vasoconstriction and tachycardia. As the syndrome progresses, hypotension and shock take over, and may be initially associated with a vagally mediated bradycardia rather than tachycardia.

The investigation and management of pre-existing pericardial effusion is outside the scope of this book. Instead we will concentrate on the identification of acute tamponade and the technique of pericardial aspiration.

Symptoms and signs of tamponade

Evidence of tamponade or impending tamponade includes dyspnoea with tachypnoea, hypotension usually with a tachycardia but occasionally with a bradycardia and pulsus parodoxus (an exaggerated fall in blood pressure of >15 mmHg on inspiration). Pulsus paradoxus may be absent in atrial fibrillation or in subjects with an atrial septal defect (ASD). A more chronic pericardial effusion may be accompanied by signs of venous congestion. The heart sounds are quiet and there may or may not be central chest pain. If there is access to the right heart, then one may observe a prominent x descent and an absent y descent. Kussmaul's sign (paradoxical jugular venous pressure (JVP)) is often absent. QRS alternans may occur – alternating large and small ECG complexes as the heart rotates within the fluid-filled pericardium. This is less common, however, and it is more likely there will be small QRS complexes present.

Unless the progression to cardiovascular collapse is rapid, the diagnosis should be confirmed by echocardiography. The presence of an echo-free space around the heart with initial diastolic collapse of the right atrium and RV free wall in the early phase and finally systolic compression are the hallmarks of tamponade.

It is very uncommon for tamponade to occur during routine diagnostic cardiac catheterization. Procedures at higher risk of tamponade include balloon valvuloplasty, electrophysiology studies, temporary pacing especially in the context of RV infarction and PCI.

Technique

The patient is connected up to the ECG monitor in the catheter lab. The first part of the procedure should be echocardiography to assess where the effusion is largest. This allows the operator to select an aspiration route that has the greatest depth of pericardial fluid and thereby minimizes perforation or laceration of coronary arteries or ventricular wall. Traditionally the subxiphoidal approach is taken, but with echo guidance may not be always the most appropriate. Other access routes may provide a better target, with the largest depth of effusion to aim at (Figure 8.8). However it is the subxiphoidal approach that is taken most often and therefore described here .The patient is then supported at 45° and the anterior wall of the lower chest and upper abdomen is washed with an antiseptic. The skin 0.5–1 cm below the xiphoid process (or access site of choice) is infiltrated with 1 per cent lignocaine (lidocaine) with a standard 21 gauge needle which is advanced until fluid is aspirated or until the hub of the needle is reached. It may be necessary to take a longer needle from a commercially available kit with more lignocaine (lidocaine) and continue to infiltrate local anaesthetic until fluid can be withdrawn. This is usually at an angle of 45° to the patient, so almost horizontal with respect to the operator (Figure 8.9). The operator should tilt the needle to the patient's left, about 45°, which directs it in line with

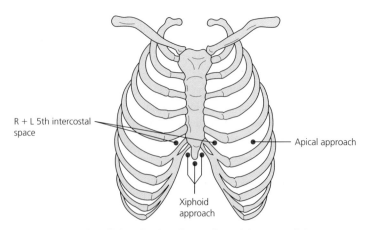

R + L 5th intercostal space

Apical approach

Xiphoid approach

Figure 8.8   Pericardial aspiration sites. Adapted from Spodick DH. *Acute Pericarditis*. New York: Grune and Stratton, 1959 and Kern MJ. *The Cardiac Catheterization Handbook*. St Louis: Mosby, 1995.

the left shoulder tip. Some operators attach an ECG lead to the base of the needle and advance until an injury current is observed. If no fluid is aspirated, then the needle should be withdrawn, flushed and reintroduced at a different angle. If the echo suggests that there is more fluid towards the apex, then this route is appropriate. The needle is kept horizontal, but directed towards the right shoulder tip. There is a higher risk of inadvertent puncture of the lung with this approach.

Once fluid is aspirated, a J-tipped wire is inserted well into the pericardial space and is seen to wrap around the heart on fluoroscopy.

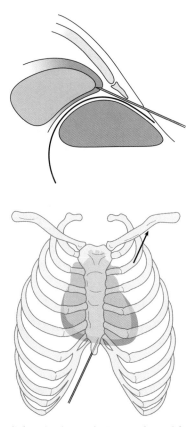

Figure 8.9 Pericardial aspiration technique. Adapted from Tilkian AG. *Cardiovascular procedures: diagnostic techniques and therapeutic procedures.* St Louis: Mosby, 1986 and Kern MJ. *The Cardiac Catheterization Handbook.* St Louis: Mosby, 1995.

A pigtail catheter is then advanced and connected up to a drainage reservoir. A rapid improvement is seen with the withdrawal of up to 200 mL of fluid, before leaving it on free drainage into a sealed reservoir. The drain needs to be fixed to the skin with non-absorbable sutures.

Effusions should be sampled and sent to the microbiology lab for Gram staining, culture and tuberculosis culture. Samples should also be sent for cytology and biochemistry. This is probably not necessary in those effusions that have occurred in the setting of a periprocedural complication in the catheter lab.

Pitfalls

Occasionally the fluid that is withdrawn looks like blood. If the needle has been connected to an ECG monitor, and no injury current was seen, then it is probably a haemorrhagic effusion. This would obviously be the case if tamponade has occurred because of a periprocedural catheter lab complication.

Occasionally it can be difficult to decide whether the catheter is in the RV or in the pericardial space on angiography or echo, especially if the tamponade is acute or traumatic and likely to be ostensibly blood based. It can be useful to inject 5 mL of saline with 0.5 mL of blood which has been agitated by passing it through a three-way tap *ex vivo* to create microbubbles. This is injected while scanning with an echocardiographic probe. The resulting bubbles will either appear in the pericardial space or in the RV. An alternative is to send a sample for blood gas analysis, which should give you a haemoglobin estimation as well. A haemorrhagic effusion as opposed to blood from the right ventricle will not clot if placed in a bowl.

WHEN TO REMOVE THE DRAIN

The fluid obviously needs to stop draining for 24 hours and then the subject can be re-echoed. If the effusion has remained absent then the drain can be removed. It needs to be removed in a manner analogous to pleural drains, as the negative intrathoracic pressure on inspiration can cause a pneumopericardium. The patient lies in a semi-recumbent position, takes a breath in and then begins to breathe out. At this point the drain is removed. The patient is asked to hold the breath at end-expiration whilst an airtight dressing is placed across the wound, to prevent air being sucked into the chest. It is worth explaining this procedure to the patient, because if it is uncomfortable, the patient may inadvertently breathe in.

Complications

Laceration of the RV free wall or either the left anterior descending (LAD) or RV branches of the right coronary artery (RCA) are the major complications. This is usually seen by a straw-coloured effusion, rapidly becoming blood stained. If this is associated with a rapid decline in haemodynamic stability then surgery is likely to be needed. Theoretically, if a coronary artery is lacerated, endovascular repair could be achieved with a covered stent. If haemodynamic collapse is progressing, the rapid evacuation of pericardial fluid and rapid intravascular fluid replacement is the only stabilizing manoeuvre, prerepair.

Other complications, such as infection, usually occur because of poor aseptic technique during insertion, poor aftercare or a line that has been left in too long.

Further reading

Ellenbogen KA. *Cardiac Pacing*. Boston: Blackwell, 1996.

References

1. Hochman JS, Boland J, Sleeper LA *et al.* Current spectrum of cardiogenic shock and effect of early revascularization on mortality. Results of an International Registry. SHOCK Registry Investigators. *Circulation* 1995; **91:** 873–881.
2. Dembitsky WP, Moore CH, Holman WL *et al.* Successful mechanical circulatory support for noncoronary shock. *J Heart Lung Transplant* 1992; **11:** 129–135.
3. Anderson RD and Gurbel PA. The effect of intra-aortic balloon counterpulsation on coronary blood flow velocity distal to coronary artery stenoses. *Cardiology* 1996; **87:** 306–312.
4. Ohman EM, Califf RM, George BS *et al.* The use of intraaortic balloon pumping as an adjunct to reperfusion therapy in acute myocardial infarction. The Thrombolysis and Angioplasty in Myocardial Infarction (TAMI) Study Group. *Am Heart J* 1991; **121:** 895–901.
5. Eltchaninoff H, Dimas AP and Whitlow PL. Complications associated with percutaneous placement and use of intraaortic balloon counterpulsation. *Am J Cardiol* 1993; **71:** 328–332.
6. Ellenbogen KA. *Cardiac Pacing*, 1st edn. Boston: Blackwell, 1992.

Catheter lab formula and formulary

Assessing cardiac output [1]

Cardiac output by Fick and modified Fick O_2 consumption method

$$CO = O_2 \text{ consumption (mL/min)}/\text{A-V}O_2 \text{ difference} \times 10$$

Where:

$$\text{A-V}O_2 \text{ difference} = \text{arterial } O_2 \text{ content} - \text{mixed venous } O_2 \text{ content}$$
$$O_2 \text{ content} = \text{saturation (\%)} \times 1.36 \times \text{Hb level (g)}$$

- Oxygen consumption should be measured using a metabolic hood, but in practice this never happens. It is normally estimated at $125 \, mL/min/m^2$.
- Mixed venous blood is normally blood from pulmonary artery.

Cardiac output by thermodilution angiography

The measurement of cardiac output by thermodilution is more commonly seen in an intensive care or coronary care unit setting rather than in the catheter lab. However, an overview will be given here, although the operator will need to be clear about the workings of the local piece of equipment.

The principle is that cardiac output is proportional to blood flow. An estimate of blood flow can be gained by injecting cool saline (room temperature or iced) from a proximal point, usually right atrium, and measuring the passage of the cooled blood/saline past a distal thermistor, usually in the pulmonary artery (PA). A complex calculation is performed, which takes account of transit time and speed of flow past the thermistor, and produces a value for cardiac output.

Pitfalls

- The saline needs to be at room temperature, so minimal handling is required to prevent warming of the saline.
- The distal thermistor part of the thermistor catheter needs to be in the PA.
- It is essential to be accurate regarding the volumes injected.
- It is important to co-ordinate injection with the equipment. Some will allow the operator to start, others will tell the operator when to inject. Inject smoothly but rapidly.
- Use at best three readings, but discount obvious outliers.
- The technique is invalid with tricuspid regurgitation (TR) and very low cardiac states, as passage past the thermistor is too slow.

Cardiac index

$$CI = CO \, (mL/min)/BSA \, (m^2)$$

Where CO is cardiac output and BSA is body surface area.

Stroke volume

$$SV = CO \text{ (mL/min)}/HR \text{ (bpm)}$$

Where CO is cardiac output and HR is heart rate.

Stroke index

$$SI = SV \text{ (mL/beat)}/BSA \text{ (m}^2)$$

Where SV is stroke volume and BSA is body surface area.

Vascular resistance

Pulmonary vascular resistance ((dyne.s)/cm^5)

$$PVR = (\text{mean PA pressure (mmHg)} - \text{PCWP (mmHg)})/CO \text{ (L/min)}$$

Where PA is pulmonary artery, PCWP is pulmonary capillary wedge pressure and CO is cardiac output.

Systemic vascular resistance ((dyne.s)/cm^5)

$$SVR = (\text{MAP (mmHg)} - \text{mean RA pressure (mmHg)})/CO \text{ (L/min)}$$

Where MAP is mean arterial pressure (=systemic diastolic pressure + (systemic systolic pressure – systemic diastolic pressure)/3), RA is right atrium and CO is cardiac output. Note: to convert to (dyne.s)/cm^5 – multiply by 80.

Assessing valve severity

Aortic stenosis

The data required for the calculation of aortic stenosis are not overly burdensome, but this is done less and less as echocardiography supersedes the usefulness of cardiac catheterization in this regard.

AORTIC VALVE AREA

$$AVA = AVF/(K \times \sqrt{\text{mean valve gradient}})$$

Where AVF is aortic valve flow and K is the Gorlin constant (44.3).

Quick aortic valve area

$$AVA = CO \text{ (L/min)}/\sqrt{\text{peak-to-peak gradient (mmHg)}}$$

This is only really valid for heart rates 60–100 bpm. Key data required:

1. Cardiac output (CO) (mL/min) – See above
2. Aortic valve flow (mL/s):

   $$AVF = CO \text{ (mL/min)}/(\text{systolic ejection period} \times HR)$$

3. Mean aortic valve gradient (mmHg).

This is usually derived by software employed by the physiology technicians. Otherwise it is a wearisome business of planimetry of the area
under the curve of the LV trace (cm^2) minus the planimetry of the aortic trace (cm^2) both bounded within the systolic ejection period. The
result is multiplied by a correction factor (i.e. how many mmHg is
represented by 1 cm on the printed trace). The result is then divided by
the systolic ejection period from the same trace in centimetres. The
computer-derived value is quicker and probably more accurate.

Mitral stenosis

The estimation of mitral valve area and mean mitral valve gradient is
quite difficult, driven in the main by difficulties gaining good-quality
simultaneous PCWP and LV traces, allowing an indirect left atrial pressure to be ascertained and then compared with direct LV pressure.
However, it will tend to overestimate mitral valve gradient, because the
phase delay in the waveforms makes alignment more difficult.

Occasionally trans-septal punctures may be necessary, but their
description is beyond the scope of this book.

MITRAL VALVE AREA

$$MVA - MVF/0.85 \times K \times \sqrt{\text{mean valve gradient}}$$

Where K is the Gorlin constant (44.3), 0.85 is the correction factor for mitral and tricuspid valve calculations and

MVF = CO (mL/min)/diastolic filling period (s) $\times$ HR (bpm)

Mean valve gradient is derived from computer data integrating the area between LA and LV pressure curves in the diastolic filling period.

Shunt calculation

Any shunt that causes mixing of blood from the right and left side of the vascular systems needs to be investigated. The diagnostic process and technique for the acquisition of blood samples is described in Chapter 6 (right heart catheterization). Any significant right to left shunt is grossly abnormal, unless it is small and seen as part of an atrial septal defect and patent foramen ovale assessment, perhaps with a Valsalva manoeuvre.

Left to right shunt

We will only describe a simplified shunt calculation by oximetry. A full saturation run fulfils two roles: to locate the first step up in saturation and therefore the location of the shunt and to allow calculation of the size of the shunt. A full saturation run should include:

- Pulmonary artery (PA) – main, left and right
- Right ventricle (RV) – high, mid and apex
- Right atrium (RA) – high, mid and low
- Superior vena cava (SVC) – high and low
- Inferior vena cava (IVC) – high and low
- Mixed arterial.

However, for calculation of a shunt, only the mixed arterial, PA, SVC and IVC need to be taken, as the pulmonary vein saturation is assumed to be 95 per cent.

The ratio of pulmonary (Qp) to systemic flow (Qs) should equal 1; any value above 1.5 suggests significant shunting from left to right and the defect may need closure.

Qp/Qs = (mixed arterial – mixed venous)/(95 – pulmonary artery)

Where mixed venous = ((3 $\times$ SVC) + IVC)/4

Pitfalls

- A small (<20 per cent) shunt may be missed.
- Patent ductus arteriosus does not produce adequate mixing in the pulmonary artery and could be missed, over- or underestimated.
- High systemic flow rates will overdetect a shunt
- Massive vasodilatation (i.e. sepsis, allergic reaction) will cause shunting.

Assessing glomerular filtration rate (GFR) by estimating creatinine clearance

$$\text{Creatinine clearance} = (1.2 \times (140 - \text{age in years}) \times \text{weight in kg})/\text{plasma creatinine}$$

For female patients the result of the formula is multiplied by 0.85; for patients who are of black ethnicity the result of the formula is multiplied by 1.18.

Catheter lab pharmacology

Anxiolytics

DIAZEPAM

Indication: On-table sedation with amnesia for acute anxiety. The duration of action is much longer than midazolam, making it less than ideal for short procedures.
Route: i.v. or p.o.
Dose: 5 mg orally or 2.5–10 mg by slow incremental intravenous injection. The dose needs to be reduced in the elderly.
Caution: Intravenous sedation mandates pulse-oximetry during the procedure, as respiratory depression and arrest are possible. Beware of second-phase sedation some hours after administration because of active metabolites.

MIDAZOLAM

Indication: Short-acting amnesic hypnotic suitable for on-table sedation for acute anxiety. Occasionally useful after major catheter lab events

to induce amnesia, and to avoid catheter lab phobias. Open discussion of complication pre and post is probably more effective.
Route: i.v. only.
Dose: 2–7.5 mg by slow intravenous injection. The dose needs to be reduced in the elderly. The effect should be titrated up, but 2.5 mg is useful for small subjects and 5 mg for larger subjects.
Caution: Intravenous sedation mandates pulse oximetry during the procedure, as respiratory depression and arrest are possible, though unusual.
Drug interaction: Verapamil and diltiazem both interfere with metabolism, leading to enhanced sedation.

TEMAZEPAM

Indication: Oral premedication.
Route: p.o. only
Dose: 20–40 mg orally (10–20 mg in the elderly).
Caution: Drowsiness.

Analgesics

DIAMORPHINE

Indication: Opioid analgesic, suitable for on-table analgesia. May cause less hypotension than morphine. Associated with significant sedation and anxiolytic effects. Sedation less than seen with benzodiazepines. This remains our anxiolytic/sedative/analgesic of choice and we use it more often than benzodiazepines even for high anxiety states.
Route: i.v. in the catheter lab.
Dose: 2.5–5 mg by slow intravenous injection. The dose needs to be reduced in the elderly.
Caution: Intravenous sedation mandates pulse oximetry during the procedure, as respiratory depression and arrest are possible.
Drug interaction: Relatively safe as an acute drug within the lab.

MORPHINE

Indication: Standard opioid analgesic, suitable for on-table analgesia. Associated with significant sedation, anxiolytic effects and vasodilatory effects.
Route: i.v. only.

Dose: 5–10 mg by slow intravenous injection. The dose needs to be reduced in the elderly. It is usually accompanied by an antiemetic.

Caution: Intravenous sedation with opiates mandates pulse oximetry during the procedure, as respiratory depression and arrest are possible.

Drug interaction: Relatively safe as an acute drug within the lab. Chronic dosing is another issue and the British National Formulary (BNF) should be consulted.

Antiarrhythmics

ADENOSINE

Indication: Diagnosis and cardioversion of tachycardia. Inducing maximal vasodilatation of the resistance arterioles in pressure and flow wire studies. Occasionally as a therapeutic manoeuvre in situations of slow/no reflow in interventional procedures.

Route: i.v. or intracoronary in the catheter lab.

Dose: 3–12 mg by rapid intravenous fusion for tachycardia diagnosis/therapy or 140 μg/kg/min by intravenous fusion in pressure wire study. This needs to be infused through a large-bore cannula in the antecubital fossa or a central vein. Intracoronary bolus dose is variable between 20 and 40 μg for the RCA and 30–60 μg for the LCA, dependent on operator.

Caution: Asthma, pre-excited atrial fibrillation (AF) (i.e. in Wolff–Parkinson–White syndrome). Heart transplantation because of excessive sensitivity to the effect of adenosine. Obviously any degree of AV block.

Drug interaction: Effect increased by dipyridamole and decreased by theophylline.

FLECAINIDE

Indication: Atrioventricular nodal reentry tachycardia (AVNRT)/atrioventricular reentry tachycardia (AVRT), acute AF, rarely ventricular tachycardia (VT).

Route: i.v. in the catheter lab.

Dose: 2 mg/kg over 10–30 minutes by slow intravenous injection. This is followed by a maintenance infusion of 1.5 mg/kg for 1 hour and then 0.1–0.25 mg/kg/hour. The cumulative dose in 24 hours should be <600 mg.

Caution: Pacemakers may have an acute increase in threshold with i.v. flecainide. High-grade AV block, the elderly. Hepatic and renal impairment.

Drug interaction: Enhanced bradycardia with beta-blockers and rate-limiting calcium channel blockers. Rare reports of asystole with verapamil.

LIGNOCAINE (LIDOCAINE)

Indication: VT.
Route: i.v. only.
Dose: 100 mg as an intravenous injection over 1–2 minutes. This is followed by a maintenance infusion of 4 mg per minute for 30 minutes, 2 mg/minute for 2 hours and 1 mg/minute thereafter.
Caution: Hypotension, as i.v. injection can cause a fall in blood pressure. Hepatic impairment. Sinus bradycardia and all grades of AV block.
Drug interaction: Increased risk of myocardial depression with other antiarrhythmics and beta-blockers.

AMIODARONE

Indication: VT, AVNRT/AVRT and acute AF.
Route: i.v. in the catheter lab.
Dose: 300 mg over 3 minutes by intravenous injection. This is followed by a maintenance infusion of 900 mg over 24 hours.
Caution: Hypotension, as i.v. injection can cause a fall in blood pressure. Hepatic impairment, although this is only really an issue with chronic oral dosing. Bradycardia.
Drug interaction: Increased risk of VT with concomitant disopyramide, procainamide and quinidine. Increased risk of bradycardia with rate-limiting calcium channel blocker and beta-blockers. It is relatively safe as an acute drug within the lab. However, chronic oral dosing is another issue and the BNF should be consulted.

Antibradycardic

ATROPINE

Indication: Bradycardia.
Route: i.v. in the catheter lab.
Dose: 0.3–1.2 mg by intravenous injection.
Caution: High-grade AV block.
Drug interaction: Relatively safe as an acute drug within the lab.

Antihypotensive

EPINEPHRINE (ADRENALINE)

Indication: Hypotension during therapeutic cardiac procedures. Works by increasing force of contraction and may have a role in the management of no flow/slow reflow after angioplasty.
Route: i.c. via guide catheter.
Dose: 5–10 μg aliquots if into aortic root or 1–2 μg if i.c. This is achieved by putting half a minijet syringe in a 500 mL bag of saline, which generates a 1 μg/mL solution. Inject slowly, especially if in the coronary artery, as VT/VF can ensue. In the management of contrast reactions 10 μg is given i.v. followed by 1–4 μg/min or 60–240 mL/h of the above solution.
Drug interactions: Arrhythmias may be more likely if halothane and enflurane are used. Tricyclic antidepressants and beta-blockers can cause an exaggerated hypertensive effect.

DOBUTAMINE

Indication: Hypotension, cardiogenic preshock and shock. Works by acting on β_1 receptors.
Route: i.v. via large-calibre peripheral line or central venous cannula.
Dose: 2.5–10 μg/kg/min.
Cautions: Drug interactions.
Drug interactions: Tricyclic antidepressants and beta-blockers can cause an exaggerated hypertensive effect.

PHENYLEPHRINE

Indication: Hypotension during therapeutic cardiac procedures. Works by increasing afterload by vasoconstriction.
Route: i.a. via femoral sheath.
Dose: 200–300 μg aliquots.

Intracoronary vasodilators

GLYCERYL TRINITRATE

Indication: Coronary artery spasm, no reflow, preintervention and pre pressure wire.
Route: i.c. via diagnostic or guiding catheter.
Dose: 100–200 μg aliquots.

ISOSORBIDE DINITRATE

Indication: Coronary artery spasm, no reflow, preintervention and pre pressure wire.
Route: i.c. via diagnostic or guiding catheter.
Dose: 1–2 mg aliquots.

VERAPAMIL

Indication: Coronary artery spasm and no reflow.
Route: i.c. via diagnostic or guiding catheter.
Dose: 100–200 µg aliquots.
Cautions: Coadministration of oral beta-blockers, second- or third-degree AV block or sinus bradycardia.

Drugs used in anaphylactoid reactions

CHLORPHENAMINE (CHLORPHENIRAMINE)

Indication: Anaphylactoid reactions.
Route: i.v. via peripheral venous cannula.
Dose: 10 mg three times daily.
Cautions: May cause drowsiness, paradoxical stimulation and anti-muscarinic effects – dry eyes and mouth.
Drug interactions: Virtually negligible.

HYDROCORTISONE

Indication: Anaphylactoid reactions.
Route: i.v. via peripheral venous cannula.
Dose: 100–200 mg four times daily.
Cautions: Systemic infections and administration in immune-compromised patients are relative contraindications in the BNF. Most side effects are due to chronic rather that acute dosing effect.
Drug interactions: Virtually negligible in the acute setting.

RANITIDINE

Indication: Severe anaphylactoid reactions, H_2 receptor blocker which works via a proposed synergistic effect on the H_1 receptor.
Route: i.v. via peripheral venous cannula over 2 minutes.
Dose: 50 mg three times daily.

Cautions: Porphyria. May cause agitation and occasionally tachycardia.
Drug interactions: Virtually negligible.

Further reading

Baim Donald S and Grossman William (eds). *Grossman's Cardiac Catheterization, Angiography, and Intervention*, 6th edn. Philadelphia: Lippincott Williams & Wilkins, 2000.
British National Formulary. British Medical Association and the Royal Pharmaceutical Society of Great Britain, 2005.
Kern MJ (ed.) *Cardiac Catheterization Handbook*, 2nd edn. St Louis: Mosby, 1995.

References

1. Kern MJ (ed.) *Cardiac Catheterization Handbook*, 2nd edn. St Louis: Mosby, 1995.

Additional angiographic material 10

In this chapter, the angiographic images that we have collected which are interesting or unusual, but which did not illustrate important points in the text are included.

Left coronary artery

Figure 10.1 shows a typical features of the muscle bridge in the left anterior descending (LAD) territory. The first panel demonstrates the artery being open in diastole. However, during left ventricular (LV) systole, the artery is compressed by muscular contraction and flow is a occluded or reduced. This only occurs if the artery is intramuscular, and epicardial arteries are not affected.

Figure 10.2 demonstrates an unusual phenomenon. In this angiographic image there is a fistula from the proximal LAD coronary artery to the main pulmonary artery. This is seen to have a number of branches and produced significant shunting of blood. This type of abnormality is

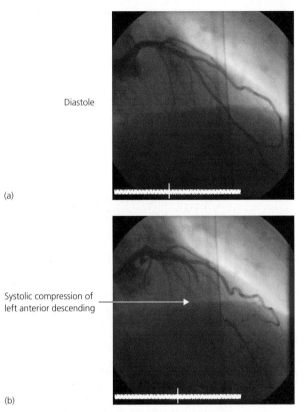

Diastole

(a)

Systolic compression of
left anterior descending

(b)

Figure 10.1 Muscle bridging in left anterior descending artery.

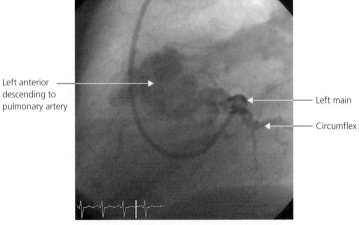

Left anterior
descending to
pulmonary artery

Left main

Circumflex

Figure 10.2 Left anterior descending to pulmonary artery fistula.

associated with a coronary steal syndrome. This was subsequently closed with multiple coils.

Figure 10.3 is a representation of the typical angiographic appearances of polyarteritis nodosa. There are distal small aneurysmal and ectatic segments of all visible coronary arteries. Polyarteritis nodosa is also a vasculitic process and occlusive coronary disease is also seen.

In this still angiographic image of a left anterior oblique (LAO) caudal view of a left coronary artery (Figure 10.4), there is marked proximal

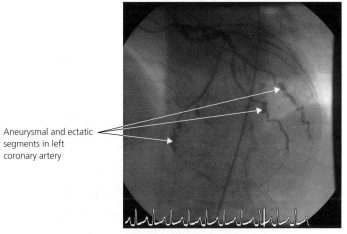

Aneurysmal and ectatic segments in left coronary artery

Figure 10.3   Left coronary artery in polyarteritis nodosa.

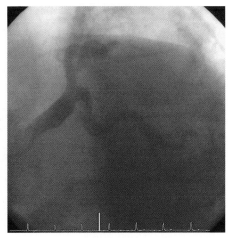

Figure 10.4   Severe coronary ectasia.

ectasia of the left main stem, LAD and circumflex arteries. The natural history of this process is uncertain, but may be linked to rapidly progressive coronary artery disease or rupture and sudden cardiac death.

In Figure 10.5 the first panel demonstrates a rupture of a circumflex coronary artery. This process can happen spontaneously, but in this example was due to a wire perforation or balloon-induced perforation during angioplasty. The second panel demonstrates contrast hold-up outside the normal coronary artery contour, which is indicative of a contained rupture of the LAD. It would be an unusual appearance for a spontaneous coronary artery dissection.

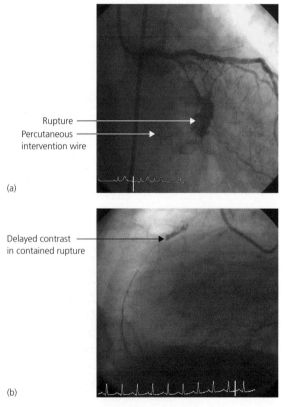

(a)

Rupture

Percutaneous intervention wire

(b)

Delayed contrast in contained rupture

Figure 10.5   Rupture of left coronary artery.

Figure 10.6 demonstrates two different types of dual LAD systems. In Figure 10.6a the LAD artery divides into two branches. The branch on the left supplies only septal arteries and produces no branches to the apex or the diagonal territory. The branch to the right-hand side of the picture produces only diagonal arteries, and no septal arteries. Figure 10.6b shows a different configuration. In this example, a small LAD continues into the ventricular groove, giving a small number of septal arteries before terminating. The diagonal artery arises and crosses out of the interventricular groove for a short period of time, where it gives off further diagonal branches. It then crosses back into the interventricular groove, to supply the apex of the ventricle.

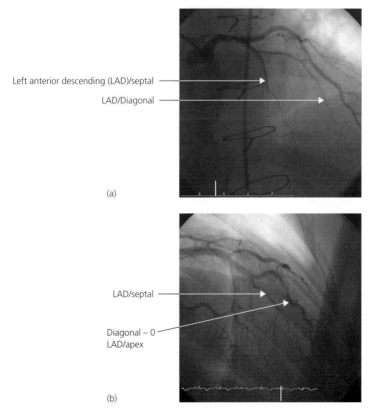

Left anterior descending (LAD)/septal

LAD/Diagonal

(a)

LAD/septal

Diagonal – 0
LAD/apex

(b)

Figure 10.6   Dual left anterior descending systems.

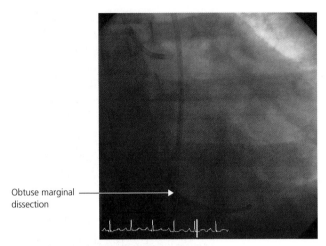

Obtuse marginal dissection

Figure 10.7   Contrast persisting in dissection.

Figure 10.7 demonstrates the persistence of contrast in the distal circumflex territory in right anterior oblique (RAO) caudal view. This shows how important it is to continue the acquisition well beyond the point where the injection phase has stopped. It is only in this situation where delayed contrast hold-up will be picked up. In this case this was a spontaneous coronary artery dissection presenting as a myocardial infarction.

Right coronary artery

Figure 10.8 shows two views in LAO of a right coronary artery (RCA). In Figure 10.8a, it can be clearly seen that there are separate origins for the main RCA and the conus branch, which is more upwardly pointing. This places it at risk of what occurs in the second panel, which is selective catheterization of this branch. In this example the catheter unfortunately plugs the RCA. This combination of poor inflow and contrast is well known to provoke ventricular fibrillation.

Figure 10.9, page 294 shows the RCA in RAO view in a patient who has presented with an acute inferior myocardial infarction. It demonstrates the original plaque, which has ruptured, leaving a cavity in the

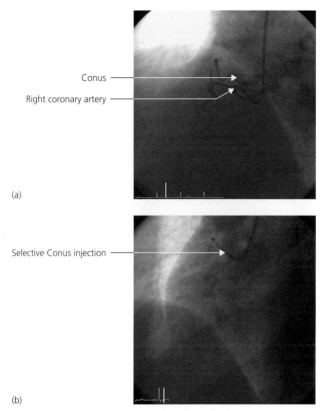

Conus

Right coronary artery

(a)

Selective Conus injection

(b)

Figure 10.8 Conus branch of right coronary artery.

mid portion. The material from within the plaque will have embolized downstream with obvious consequences.

Figure 10.10 is an example of an anomalous RCA origin. This is perhaps the most common anomalous origin for the RCA, where it arises from the junction of right and left coronary sinuses, just below the sinotubular junction. It is often easier to engage the ostium of this anomalous vessel from the left coronary sinus with gentle clockwise torque on the catheter to move it from left to right coronary sinus. Catheters that may prove useful will include Amplatz left (AL)0.75, AL1, modified Amplatz right or Williams catheter.

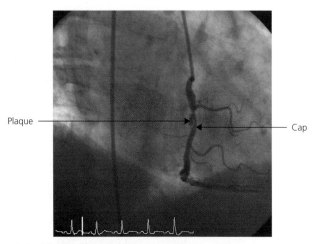

Plaque ———

——— Cap

Figure 10.9   Right coronary artery ruptured plaque.

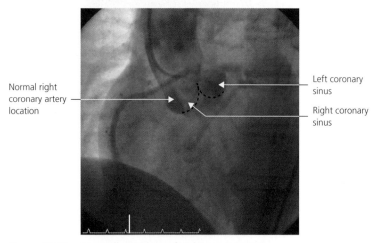

Normal right
coronary artery
location

Left coronary
sinus

Right coronary
sinus

Figure 10.10   Anomalous origin of right coronary artery.

Left ventricle

Figure 10.11a shows a dilated LV cavity, taken during diastole. However, Figure 10.11b, which is taken in peak systole, clearly demonstrates that the anterior, anterior apical and apical segments are akinetic.

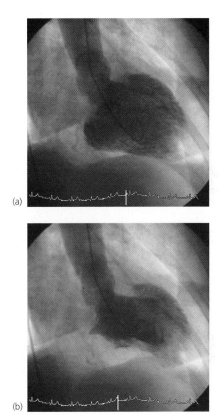

(a)

(b)

Figure 10.11 Left ventricular anterior akinesia.

Figure 10.12 are two further examples of LV abnormalities. Figure 10.12a shows an end diastolic image of the LV cavity, which clearly demonstrates apical and anteroapical calcification. Figure 10.12b is difficult to discern from a still image, but the apical aneurysm is marked and the original LV cavity is highlighted by dashed lines.

Figure 10.13, page 297 is a beautiful example of a sinus of Valsalva aneurysm. This presented a lot of difficulty selectively engaging the left coronary artery. An MRI image clearly demonstrates the location and extent of the aneurysm.

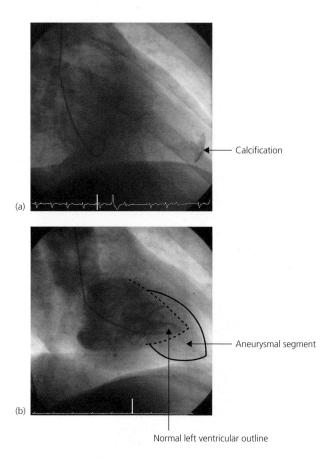

Figure 10.12   Apical left ventricular calcification and aneurysm.

Radial artery

Figure 10.14 shows two complications associated with the radial route for cardiac catheterization. Figure 10.14a shows the problems with a previous radial procedure, where the radial artery has subsequently occluded. Interestingly, it can be seen that despite the radial occlusion,

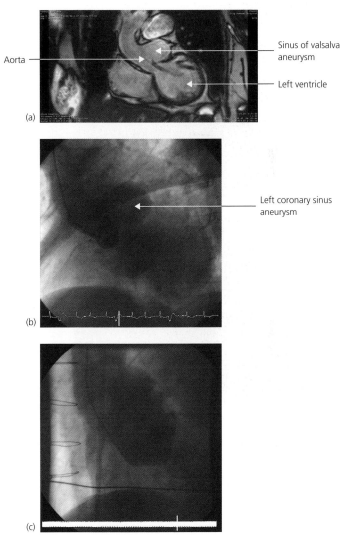

(a)

Aorta

Sinus of valsalva aneurysm

Left ventricle

(b)

Left coronary sinus aneurysm

(c)

Figure 10.13 Sinus of Valsalva aneurysm.

collateralization to the palmar arcade is still clearly visible. Figure 10.14b shows one of the reasons why it is not possible to categorize every patient from the radial route. This patient had an asymptomatic right subclavian artery occlusion.

298 ADDITIONAL ANGIOGRAPHIC MATERIAL

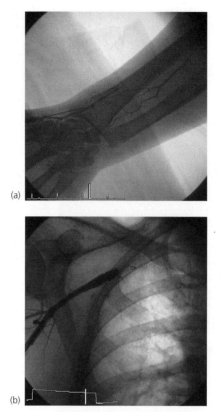

(a)

(b)

Figure 10.14 Occluded radial artery and subclavian stenosis.

Femoral artery

Figure 10.15 demonstrates three complications with the femoral route. Figure 10.15a demonstrates a tortuous femoral and iliac artery. This is more commonly seen in patients who have peripheral vascular disease or longstanding hypertension. The difficulty can sometimes be overcome by using a long femoral sheath or a Judkins R4 catheter with a slippy Terumo wire in order to negotiate the tortuous segment. A double length exchange wire should be used when access to the aortic root has been achieved.

Figure 10.15b shows a chronic aortic dissection, which was revealed after a failed attempt to cannulate the right femoral artery, and

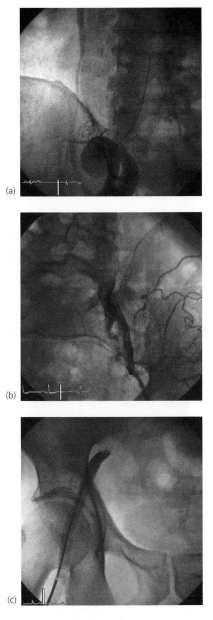

Figure 10.15 Iliac tortuosity, dissection and kinked sheath.

subsequent successful puncture of the left. Inability to advance the wire cleanly provoked a left femoral angiogram. This shows a chronic dissection affecting the aortic bifurcation and iliac artery.

Figure 10.15c shows an occluded common iliac artery.

Renal angiography

Figure 10.16 demonstrates renal angiography performed as part of a cardiac catheterization procedure. Figure 10.16a shows a left renal artery stenosis and Figure 10.16b shows a right renal artery stenosis. We initially felt there was also a pelviureteric junction obstruction, but on

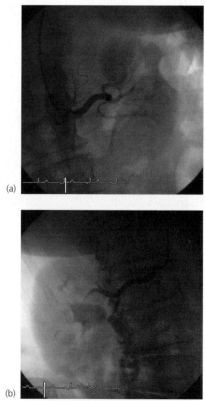

(a)

(b)

Figure 10.16 Renal artery stenosis.

discussing it with our radiology colleagues, they felt this probably represented normal ureteric peristalsis.

Vein graft angiography

Figure 10.17 demonstrates a 15-year-old vein graft to an obtuse marginal vessel. This vein graft is degenerate and has disease over 50 per cent of its length. In other views the disease appears more significant than in this picture, but this image demonstrates the length of the diseased segment. You can also see that the run-off into the graft is also poor.

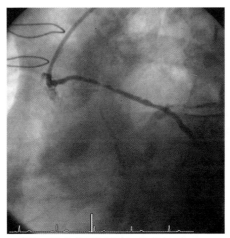

Figure 10.17   Degenerate saphenous vein bypass graft to obtuse marginal artery.

Index

Bold page number refer to figures and *italic* page numbers indicate tables.